MEDS, INC.

Excellence in Nursing Education

Successful Problem-Solving and Test-Taking for Nursing and NCLEX-RN Exams:

Easy Steps to Passing

Fourth Edition

Author:
Patricia A. Hoefler, R.N., M.S.N.

Contributing Author:
Jennifer Burks, R.N., M.S.N.

Medical Education Development Services, Inc.
P.O. Box 4520
Silver Spring, Maryland 20914

Senior Editor:	Amelia R. Hummel
Editors:	Chellis E. Neal, R.N., B.A., J.D.
	Kathleen Lynch
Design Coordinator:	Kathleen Lynch

Fourth Edition, ©1995.

Copies of this book may be obtained from:
Medical Education Development Services, Inc.
P.O. Box 4520
Silver Spring, Maryland 20914
(301) 622-9191

ISBN: 1-56533-013-7

Printed in the United States of America.

Table of Contents

CHAPTER	PAGE
i. Introduction	i
1. How to Use This Book	1
2. Your Personalized Study Program for Nursing Exams	5
3. How Do I Avoid "Reading Into" the Question?	11
4. How Do I Choose Between the Two Best Options?	31
5. Learning to Answer Communication Questions	45
6. Learning to Answer Questions that Select Priorities	57
7. Learning to Answer Questions that Involve Use of the Nursing Process	67
8. How to Take a Timed Nursing Exam	89
9. How to Prepare for the NCLEX-RN Exam	95
10. A Final Exam	117
11. Answers and Analysis	131
Additional Study Materials for NCLEX Candidates	163
Special Tips for Using the Companion Computer Disk	164

Introduction

Q

Why a Book on Problem-Solving and Test-Taking for Nursing Exams?

A

The purpose of this book is to help you master the test-taking skills needed to do well on your nursing course exams and, ultimately, on the NCLEX-RN Exam and other professional nursing examinations.

The material in this book is important because test-taking has become an essential professional skill.

The problem-solving and analytical skills discussed in these materials are useful throughout nursing school, for the NCLEX-RN Exam, and throughout your nursing career.

Test-taking is not presently taught in most nursing programs. This book was written to fill a gap in the standard nursing curriculum. Written by a nurse educator with well over a decade of grass-roots experience in presenting NCLEX review courses and test-taking seminars across the U.S. and Canada, *Successful Problem-Solving and Test-Taking* addresses your needs as a nursing student and NCLEX candidate, and its methods respect the nursing profession. The test-taking guidelines and strategies in this book will help you to look at test questions from a different perspective. With training and practice you'll find in this book, you can become more analytical and a better problem-solver!

Since you began taking nursing courses, have you heard yourself making the following comments?:

"I do very well clinically, but when it comes to the nursing exams I do poorly. Why are the questions so hard?"

"I get excellent grades clinically, but the scores on my nursing exams decrease my overall grade in nursing."

"I study very hard, but my nursing exam grades do not show it because the test questions are so confusing. Why don't the instructors learn to write clearer test questions so that I can answer them?"

The NCLEX-RN Exam, of course, presents additional challenges. If you are getting ready to take the NCLEX-RN Exam, are you nervous about preparing for it? Are you and your fellow students asking yourselves:

"How can I possibly review all my nursing content before the exam?"

"What's the computerized NCLEX-RN like? And how do I know that I will get a fair selection of questions with the new computerized adaptive testing?"

"Is there any way to practice answering NCLEX-type questions before I take the exam?"

If you find nursing exams difficult, you are not alone! Like many other nursing students, you probably find taking multiple choice nursing examinations a stressful experience. But nursing exams -- even the NCLEX -- don't have to be quite so stressful or worrisome!

Research has demonstrated that regardless of how similar the educational background and training of any two students may be, the test-wise candidate will score higher, on average, than the less skilled test-taker every time.

This is also true for nursing exams. Learning how to effectively prepare for an exam and improving your test-taking skills will **decrease test-taking anxiety** and enable you to **make the most of your nursing knowledge** when answering test questions. This book is dedicated to helping you do just that. With *Successful Problem-Solving and Test-Taking,* you can improve your score on nursing exams and on the NCLEX-RN!

Q Why Are Nursing Exams So Difficult?

A

Today's nursing students are highly motivated, very capable students. Before entering nursing school, some of you may even have earned a degree in another field. Many R.N. candidates already have some working experience in the health care field. Regardless of their academic and professional background, most nursing students find nursing exams to be very different from other exams they have taken -- and very difficult. Why are nursing exams so hard?

Nursing exams are difficult because the questions ask you to make judgments and apply information -- not just recall facts.

No matter how hard you study or how much information you can recall, you will not pass unless you can apply your nursing knowledge and make good nursing judgments on the exam.

Another reason nursing exams seem difficult is because the questions are written at what nurse educators refer to as a "high cognitive level." In other words, the questions seem difficult because they are designed to be difficult to answer! The complex questions on nursing exams are designed to test problem-solving and critical thinking skills as well as mastery of the nursing content. As part of preparing you to become a professional nurse, these exams must assess your ability to **identify problems in clinical situations, apply nursing principles, set nursing priorities, and evaluate nursing care.** The questions are complex because such decisions are **rarely black and white.**

Q Why Do I Suddenly Need New Test-Taking Skills?

A

Multiple choice testing is here to stay, in nursing courses and in professional certification at all levels. The NCLEX has developed its own distinctive characteristics because the nursing profession is so specialized. Many nursing course exams now use questions similar to those on the NCLEX and other professional examinations to better prepare students for the NCLEX. Every nursing student, therefore, needs specialized test-taking skills **to be able to correctly interpret and answer the unique kinds of questions found on nursing exams.**

Have you had trouble selecting the correct answer to questions that present a clinical scenario and ask you to "identify the sign or symptom to which the nurse would give immediate attention?" Or have you found it confusing when asked to "select the highest (or lowest) priority nursing intervention" in a certain clinical scenario? Such questions are asking you to problem-solve. In nursing, problem-solving entails figuring out what the nurse should (or shouldn't) do when providing care to a client. Many nursing students find it hard to understand these questions.

Sometimes a question may present so much information about a clinical situation that it may be difficult to determine which factors are most important. Or a question may seem to have two, three, or even four correct answers. Although students often regard such questions as "trick" questions, they are actually using a special kind of test-taking logic.

> **In a clinical situation, many actions might be appropriate. On an exam only one will be the best or priority action. This is how the exam tests your nursing judgment as well as your nursing knowledge. It is very important to know how to go about answering judgment questions!**

You also need new skills because you need to be prepared to answer the many **different questions** that relate to a given clinical area. For example, there may be communication questions in addition to questions about pathophysiology, medications, and nursing interventions and their rationales. These questions are included because therapeutic communication is so important in the safe and effective practice of nursing. An exam designed to test your knowledge in a specific clinical area will, therefore, be likely to include communication questions involving that area. Sometimes NCLEX-RN candidates report finding a great many 'psych' questions on the NCLEX, many of which were really communication questions. There are similar questions that test your ability to do client teaching. You need to be able to identify these questions and know what they are really about!

Other questions testing your nursing knowledge may be focused on safety or infection control, or on providing care to infants and children, pregnant clients and new mothers, elderly clients, clients with sensory impairments, confused clients, or other clients with special needs. On nursing exams, you may be called upon to apply your knowledge of everything from body mechanics to growth and development to special diets. This is especially true on the NCLEX.

For these reasons, you need to know how to prepare for exams that use such a comprehensive approach. You need to know how to answer all these special types of questions. In addition to reviewing nursing content, your preparation for either a course exam or the NCLEX should include a plan for improving your test-taking skills and practice in answering problem-solving questions. *Successful Problem-Solving and Test-Taking* will show you how to plan your review and how to answer the difficult questions you will find on your exams.

Q: Will This Book Help Me Become a Better Nurse?

A: **Yes!** Questions on nursing exams are written at a high cognitive level because they use the nursing process. *Successful Problem-Solving and Test-Taking* is designed specifically for nursing students. It continually emphasizes the nursing process because this is the process by which nurses apply their nursing knowledge and make clinical decisions.

As you will see in Chapter Two, "Your Personalized Study Program for Nursing Exams," your comprehensive review for a nursing exam will need to include, among other things, early and late signs and symptoms, pathophysiology, medications, treatments, side and adverse effects, complications, client teaching, diet, comfort and safety measures, infection control, and other specific nursing measures. In the vocabulary of the nursing process, you will need to know how to assess a client and analyze data, how to plan nursing care, and how to implement and evaluate that care. You also need to know how to prioritize, how to assess safety risks, and how to communicate therapeutically. You need to know these things not just to answer test questions, but also to be an effective nurse. The same approach is used in reviewing nursing content for the NCLEX.

Nursing educators believe that testing is an essential component of the learning process. The nurse educators at MEDS, Inc., are convinced that improved methods of reviewing nursing content and learning problem-solving skills enhances critical thinking ability -- not only on exams but also in clinical situations, where it counts the most!

Q What Will I Get Out Of This Book?

A

The good news is that becoming a test-wise nursing student or NCLEX candidate is a skill you can learn! *Successful Problem-Solving and Test-Taking* is the only nursing test-taking manual that teaches a unique, specialized three-step method for correctly interpreting test questions. This method was developed through many years of grass-roots experience teaching NCLEX review courses and nursing exam test-taking workshops, and it has enabled thousands of nursing students throughout the United States and Canada to increase their exam scores and to pass the NCLEX on their first try. *Successful Problem-Solving and Test-Taking* unlocks the mysteries of the unique **"test-taking logic"** of nursing exams, including the NCLEX. It shows you how to decode the questions and how to decide between possible options when you are not sure of the answer. This book gives you essential techniques for correctly interpreting nursing test questions and criteria to use in selecting your answer.

Because this book is designed to help you master nursing exams and, most importantly, the NCLEX-RN Exam, the test-taking techniques presented in the *Successful Problem-Solving and Test-Taking* book use the nursing process. They are designed to enhance and polish your professional problem-solving and critical thinking skills. In addition, the study and review techniques presented should yield a definite payoff in the area of time-management, which is a critical issue for so many of today's nursing students.

If you are an NCLEX candidate, you need to become familiar with the unique NCLEX format. You also need to practice using the strategies required to answer certain kinds of nursing questions. Chapter Nine in *Successful Problem-Solving and Test-Taking* will give you the **"inside scoop"** on the NCLEX-RN, answering all your questions about the exam and addressing your concerns. **"How can I review all the clinical areas, and how long will it take?" "Will I run out of time**

on the NCLEX?" "How do I keep from 'reading into' a question?" "What kind of an answer is this question looking for?" "How can I choose between the two best options when both appear correct?" "What should I do when I'm just not sure of the answer?" This book explains it all!

Be sure to note the special features of *Successful Problem-Solving and Test-Taking* that are provided for maximum learning. **The drills in each chapter and the "Final Exam" in Chapter Ten let you practice your new test-taking skills and assess your progress. Chapter Eleven provides complete rationales for all the correct and incorrect options in each question.**

Finally, the **computer diskette** provided with this book offers you the opportunity to become familiar with the screen design and special format of the computerized NCLEX Exam. We strongly recommend that you take advantage of this special option!

We invite you to view this presentation as a coaching session by an expert nurse educator who will offer you suggestions and guidelines. Nursing students and nurse educators, as well as NCLEX-RN candidates, will find this new and fresh approach extremely helpful. Here, finally, is a book with an easy-to-follow approach to showing you how to **make the most of your nursing knowledge** on nursing exams. We are confident that this book will give you the skills you need to improve your test scores and "ace" the NCLEX. We hope you will enjoy *Successful Problem-Solving and Test-Taking.*

Patricia A. Hoefler

Patricia A. Hoefler, R.N., M.S.N.
Program Director
MEDS, Inc.

Chapter 1

How to Use This Book

Successful Problem-Solving and Test-Taking is specifically designed to teach you the specialized skills you need to maximize your scores on nursing course exams and the NCLEX-RN Exam.

This book will show you how to:

- ☑ Correctly interpret a multiple choice nursing test question by using a quick 3-step method.
- ☑ Use test-taking strategies to eliminate distractors and select the correct answer when you are unsure.
- ☑ Apply specific guidelines to answer the special kinds of questions you are certain to find on your exams: communication questions, questions that select priorities, and questions that use the nursing process.
- ☑ Learn and practice problem-solving skills.
- ☑ Plan your review of the nursing content to be covered for the NCLEX or your nursing course exam.
- ☑ Pace yourself on a timed exam.
- ☑ Answer questions using the computerized NCLEX-RN format.

Whether you are a nursing student preparing for a course exam or a nursing graduate preparing for the NCLEX-RN Exam, we recommend that you take a few moments to familiarize yourself with the format of this book.

First, if you have not yet done so, we recommend that you go back and read the **Introduction,** "Why a Book on Problem-Solving and Test-Taking for Nursing Exams?" The Introduction includes some useful information about the different kinds of questions used on nursing exams, and will help you to understand what *Successful Problem-Solving and Test-Taking* is designed to do for you. Then, look over the **Table of Contents** for an overview of the book's overall plan.

Nursing students should read **Chapter Two,** "Your Personalized Study Program for Nursing Exams." This will show you how to review material and prepare for a nursing exam. If you are a nursing graduate, turn instead to **Chapter Nine,** "How to Prepare for the NCLEX." These two chapters will explain how to plan your review and how to use practice test questions. You may wish to read **Chapter Two** or **Chapter Nine** quickly now, to provide a context for learning the test-taking techniques and strategies in **Chapters Three** through **Seven,** and then return and read them in greater detail when you are actually planning your review. For now, be sure to note that the study methods outlined for both the NCLEX and nursing course exams incorporate the nursing process.

Next, we recommend that you read **Chapters Three** through **Seven** carefully, in detail, and in the order that they occur in the book. These are the chapters on test-taking strategies. The first is **Chapter Three,** "How Do I Avoid "Reading Into" a Test Question?" Students "read into" a test question because they are not able to interpret it correctly. This chapter explains how a test question is constructed and explains the unique "test-question logic" used in nursing exams. This chapter is the most basic and the most important of the chapters on test-taking strategies.

Chapter Four, "How Do I Choose Between the Two Best Options?" shows you how to use three powerful strategies for choosing the best option when two or more options appear equally correct, or when you aren't sure of the answer using your nursing knowledge alone. There is only one best option in each question. These strategies will help you to identify it!

Haven't you sometimes wondered what is being tested in communication questions? There are several pitfalls you need to know how to avoid in answering them! **Chapter Five,** "Learning to Answer Communication Questions," provides useful insights into what makes these questions tick and gives you some simple guidelines to follow when selecting your answer.

"What should the nurse do first?" "What is the priority nursing action at this time?" The answer depends on the clinical scenario, on what the question is asking, and on what is presented in the options from which you are to select. **Chapter Six,** "Learning to Answer Questions that Select Priorities," will show you how to apply four different priority-setting guidelines to test questions, including Maslow's Hierarchy of Needs. This chapter is ESSENTIAL for your success on the NCLEX. If you are a nursing student, learn these guidelines now and use them on your course exams. Priority-setting questions don't have to be confusing!

Chapter Seven, "Learning to Answer Questions that Use the Nursing Process," focuses on the nursing process as a problem-solving and test-taking guideline, and on key words in test questions that are signals to apply the nursing process when selecting your answer. This chapter is vital for NCLEX candidates and also can save you a lot of trouble on your nursing course exams.

When taking a timed exam, it is important to pace yourself so that you will have time to complete the exam without undue stress and without getting marooned on any one question. In **Chapter Eight,** "How to Take a Timed Nursing Exam," you will learn how to use a simple pacing method and how to use sets of practice questions to increase your test-taking speed. NCLEX candidates also will benefit from this chapter, because there is a time limit on the NCLEX and because good pacing reduces stress and improves concentration. Using a pacing technique when answering practice questions helps build speed, polish test-taking technique, and increases confidence.

Preparing for the NCLEX can be overwhelming! **Chapter Nine,** "How to Prepare for the NCLEX," gives you a simple outline to follow in designing your review and explains the best way to study. This chapter also explains how to use practice questions in your review.

When you have completed the chapters on test-taking strategies, be sure to take the Final Exam in Chapter Ten. The same exam is also provided on the enclosed computer diskette, so you have your choice of format.

Try the computerized format on your home PC or in your learning lab. It includes an automatic Personal Performance Analysis, which will show how well you are doing in interpreting test questions, using test-taking strategies, applying prioritizing guidelines, using the nursing process, answering communication questions, and demonstrating your knowledge in each of the clinical areas.

Chapter Eleven, "Answers and Analysis," provides complete rationales for each correct and incorrect answer to every question in the Final Exam. These complete rationales are hallmarks of MEDS, Inc., and are included for maximum learning. Test-taking tips are also provided. In the post-test segment on the diskette, the program "remembers" which option you chose for each question and then lets you view rationales for each correct or incorrect option. The written exam format also includes complete rationales; they are shown in **Chapter Eleven.**

This brief guided tour of *Successful Problem-Solving and Test-Taking* should give you a good idea of what you will learn and how you can use it. To begin, turn to **Chapter Two** (for nursing students) or **Chapter Nine** (for NCLEX candidates). Whether you are studying this book in a nursing class or on your own, you are already well on your way to improving your scores on nursing exams and passing the NCLEX on your first try!

Chapter 2

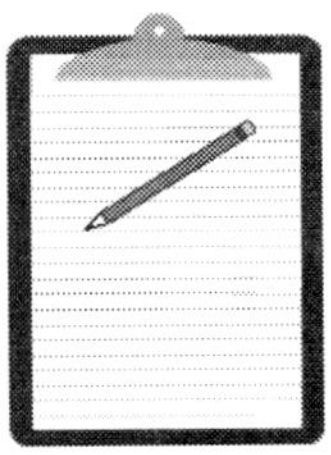

Your Personalized Study Program for Nursing Exams

Isn't it true that you begin your preparation for a nursing exam on the first day of class? After all, don't you usually review your class notes when you review for the exam? You are anticipating the exam when you take notes and ask questions in class, and when you read assigned chapters in your textbook. By planning to use good preparation, note-taking, and review techniques, you can save time and be more successful.

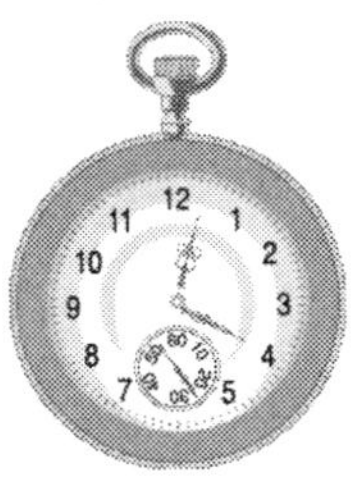

Time Management: Preparing for Class

Students today are very busy, and many complain that they never have time to read the text ahead of time. It is very important, however, to prepare for class. Even if you have only a few minutes to spend on preparation, a little preparation will go a long way to increase your understanding of the material.

Preparation will pay off in terms of better comprehension and time you will save later. In fact, studies have shown that it can cut your study time in half. So be sure to prepare!

❶ First, **skim the chapter and read the subheadings,** to get an overview of what is being covered. Then, **look at any charts or illustrations and read the captions.** Certainly you can plan to do at least this much before class!

❷ Try to **allow yourself the time to read the chapter through once, quickly. Look for basic concepts and the most important information. Make note of any questions** you may have. Your goal as you prepare for class is **understanding the material, not memorizing it.**

❸ Reading quickly and trying to get a good overview of the material will save you time now and it will improve your memory and your comprehension. This important principle is the foundation of expensive "speed-reading" courses you may have seen advertised. Try it -- it works!

❹ When you have finished your first reading, look again at the subheadings and illustrations. This will reinforce the structure of the presentation of the material and refresh your memory of what information you have covered.

How to Take Notes in Class

Your nursing instructor, in presenting material, is trying to make the material easier to understand. The instructor will, therefore, include explanations and clarifications of concepts and information covered in your textbook. When taking notes, your object should also be to **clarify.** Here are some basic principles:

❶ Always be sure you know what is being discussed. This may seem obvious, but it isn't always simple to describe the subject of a discussion. Here are some possible topics related to the study of a medical problem:

- Incidence
- Pathophysiological process
- Manifestations
- Side effects and adverse effects of treatments
- Complications
- Nursing interventions, including prioritizing
- Client teaching

❷ Be sure you understand the rationale for a treatment or intervention. Your objective here is understanding. Although you can return to the textbook later for the details, **be sure to ask a question if there is something that you don't understand.** Keep in mind that if something is not clear to you, it is probably unclear to others as well -- especially if you have prepared for the class. Asking a question can decrease your study time by half!

❸ Make sure you understand the priorities. What is most important? One clue would be any visual aids that the instructor uses, such as charts, illustrations, or notes written on the board.

❹ **Be alert for the answers to any questions you may have had while reading the assigned material.** If you have a question that is not answered during the course of the instructor's presentation, take the opportunity to ask it. Never leave a classroom if you are unclear about the information!

❺ When you are taking notes, stay focused on the topic and try to be analytical. Note-taking is not the same as taking dictation! **You should not be trying to write down everything that the instructor says. If you have a lot of difficulty following the instructor, try bringing a tape recorder instead of trying to write everything down.**

❻ **After class, preferably the same day or the next, look over your class notes and the assigned textbook material again,** quickly, and re-read any difficult sections of the text. Write down any remaining questions you have, and be sure to ask the instructor.

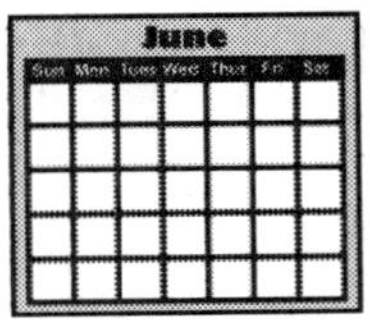

Reviewing for the Exam

Now it's exam time! You have your class notes and your textbook. How are you going to study for the exam?

Don't wait until the last minute! Take a calendar and plan what you will do to review, how long it will take and exactly when you will do it. All the leaders of the Fortune 500 use personalized written plans for important projects. Putting your plan in writing is like writing your own personal guarantee of success! So write out your plan. Then set aside the time, and plan other activities so that you will be able to make good use of your study time. If possible, plan to do your reviewing in the library, or anywhere you can be sure that you will not be interrupted. See Appendix A for MEDS, Inc's detailed study plan calendar for the NCLEX-RN Exam.

Here is a comprehensive, time-saving way to review:

❶ **Review your class notes,** paying special attention to rationales for interventions. If any are unclear, look them up in your text. As you review the material, keep in mind the phases of the **nursing process:** What should the nurse **assess**? How should the nurse **analyze** the assessment data? How should the nurse **plan** care for the client? What should the nurse keep in mind when **implementing** care? How should the nurse monitor and **evaluate** the client's response to therapy? Again, your focus is on **understanding,** so try to use your own words.

❷ **Look through the textbook. You may wish to make a brief, one-page outline of the subject, noting any areas that are particularly difficult for you.** Are you familiar with the main points? Do you understand the charts and illustrations? Reread any sections that you found unclear. If you complete your preparation ahead of time and have questions about the material, **ask your instructor!**

3. **Use some of the reviewing aids that are available in your bookstore or learning lab.** For example, MEDS, Inc. publishes a complete set of audio tapes and video tapes for the review of all clinical areas, plus special topics such as pharmacology and safety. These tapes are especially useful when reviewing for final exams, when a great deal of material is to be covered at one time. More information about these materials is available from MEDS, Inc.

4. **Use practice questions.** This is extremely important! **Practice questions assess and reinforce what you have learned.** Practice questions reflect what goes on in the real world in clinical situations, and they help you to become more analytical.

5. Teamwork harnesses brainpower -- so **study in teams with other good students if you can.** Group study is good for morale, too!

Using Practice Questions

Be sure to plan time during your review to **answer practice questions** covering the subject.

> **Answering practice questions is as important as going over your notes or reviewing your text, because it gives you a chance to practice applying your newly acquired nursing knowledge.**

As a rule of thumb, MEDS, Inc., recommends that you plan to answer about 200 practice questions in preparation for a typical 50-question exam. You will find "Q&A" (question and answer) books in your bookstore, as well as in your learning lab or library. Computerized practice tests are also available. MEDS, Inc., publishes Q&A books and software, and also offers a series of Q&A review audio tapes. When answering questions, be sure to time yourself and practice **pacing** yourself (see Chapter Eight, "How to Take a Timed Nursing Exam").

To assess your knowledge and your test-taking skills, be sure to check your answers and read the rationales! Assess the reason why you missed any questions that you answered incorrectly. Did you misunderstand or "read into" the question? Did you lack the required nursing knowledge to answer the question? Is there a test-taking strategy that would have helped you to select the correct answer?

Finally, when you have completed a set of practice questions, you may wish to return to your textbook or class notes and review any information that gave you difficulty. You may also wish to return to *Successful Problem-Solving and Test-Taking* to review how to answer particular types of questions, or how to use certain test-taking strategies.

The Payoff!

Following these guidelines for organized, streamlined preparation and review will pay off in increased confidence, increased understanding, better use of your time, and increased test scores. Try it and see!

NOTES

Chapter 3

How Do I Avoid "Reading Into" the Question?

It seems justified to lose points on an exam because you did not know the necessary information. It is extremely frustrating, however, to score poorly on an exam because you "read into" or misread the questions!

You can maximize your score on your nursing course exams and the NCLEX-RN Exam by learning some test-taking techniques and strategies. This chapter will show you some techniques to help you to read and interpret test questions correctly, and to help you eliminate incorrect options. It will also show you how to avoid the common errors made when students misread a question, and give you some helpful test-taking tips.

Three test-taking techniques are described in this chapter:

1. First, you will learn a technique for analyzing a test question by separating what the **case scenario** in the question **tells** you, from what the **stem** of the question **asks.**
2. Second, you will learn a technique for interpreting a test question by identifying the **four critical elements.**
3. Third, you will learn a technique for **eliminating incorrect options**. Each time you answer a test question, you should use **all three** of these techniques!

TECHNIQUE #1

IDENTIFYING THE "CASE SCENARIO" AND THE "STEM"

The first step in analyzing a test question is to separate what the question **tells** you from what it is **asking**.

Each test question basically consists of three parts:

1. It presents a **case scenario** statement.
2. It contains a **stem,** which asks you to select an answer.
3. It presents **four options,** from which you must select the answer.

The **case scenario** in a test question is a statement that gives you information about a clinical problem. The **stem** of a question asks you to solve a specific problem and select one of the **four options** as the answer.

Here is a sample test question set up like a computerized NCLEX-RN screen showing the **case scenario,** the **stem** and the **four options.**

Case Scenario

Stem

On the psychiatric unit a nurse observes a client standing at the window in her room and touching the glass. She also mutters to herself from time to time.

Which comment by the nurse indicates the best understanding of the client's behavior?

1. "Why are you standing by the window and touching the glass?"
2. "There you are. I came to see if you wanted to see the video we are showing on the unit?"
3. "What are you looking at throught the window?
4. "Are you hearing voices or seeing things?

Four Options

As you can see, this question **tells** you about the client's health problem. The **case scenario** in the question **gives you the clinical information** you should consider in answering the question.

The **stem** is the portion of the test question that **asks** the nurse to solve a specific problem and select one of the **four options.** The **stem** in the question **asks** you to choose the option that presents the best rationale for increasing Vitamin C in the client's diet.

The **stem** usually comes **after** the **case scenario** and asks you a question referring to the case scenario statement. Here is another sample test question with the stem in bold print:

> A client had a cerebral vascular accident two weeks ago. He is paralyzed on the left side. While getting him out of bed to sit in a wheelchair, **which nursing action is essential?**

Note that the case scenario and the stem are not always in separate sentences! Sometimes the case scenario seems to "run into" or "overlap" the stem, as it does in the above question. When this happens, you can still separate what the question is **telling** you from what it is specifically **asking**. It may be helpful in a question like this to restate the question in your own words. Here is the question restated and, again, the **stem** is in bold print:

> A client had a cerebral vascular accident two weeks ago. He is paralyzed on the left side. The nurse must get him out of bed so that he can sit in a wheelchair. **Which nursing action is essential in making such a transfer?**

Now here is another question about the same client, with the **case scenario** in bold print:

> **A client had a cerebral vascular accident two weeks ago. He is paralyzed on the left side. In transferring him to a wheelchair, the nurse notices a reddened area on his left hip.** Which nursing action is essential?

Notice that, although the stem still asks you to select an essential nursing action, the **case scenario** has been changed. It is very important to **read all the information in the introductory statement!** The second question about the client will have a different answer from the first question.

It is important to identify what the question *tells* you and what it *asks,* because:

❶ Incorrect options may "answer" something that is not actually being asked;
❷ Incorrect options may assume information that was not given in the case scenario.
❸ Reading each question carefully will help you make the most of your nursing knowledge!

NOTE➤ Some questions may not describe a specific clinical situation. For example, a question without a case scenario statement might simply ask you to select the option that best:

- identifies a sign or symptom of a specific disease.
- describes the difference between two diseases.
- identifies a sign of a problem.
- specifies the priority nursing action for a certain kind of situation.

You can think of a question **without a case scenario** statement as giving you a **subject with stem.** The stem of such a question asks you something regarding that subject.

Here is a sample test question set up like the computerized NCLEX-RN screen showing the **subject with stem,** and the **four options.**

Subject with Stem	Four Options
Remotivation therapy is used in long-term care facilities for which of the following reasons?	**1. Stimulate and encourage social participation.** **2. Reorient clients with cognitive problems.** **3. Share memories of past experiences and events.** **4. Resolve emotional problems.**

TECHNIQUE #2

IDENTIFYING THE FOUR CRITICAL ELEMENTS

Learning to identify the critical elements in a test question is crucial to interpreting the question correctly. To clarify a question's meaning, it is necessary to identify each of these elements.

The four critical elements in each test question are:

1. The **key words**.
2. The **client**.
3. The **issue**.
4. The **type of stem**.

1. What are the *key words?*

The key words are the important words or phrases in a question. Key words focus your attention on crucial ideas in the stem and in the options. Here are some phrases from questions with the key words in **bold** print:

- **early** or **late** signs
- **immediately** after surgery or in the **postoperative** period
- the **most likely** or **least likely** characteristics to occur
- the **initial** nursing action
- **after several days**
- **on the day of** admission

It's important to be able to recognize **key words** because a common type of distractor is a statement that would be correct if the **key words** were missing or different. For instance, a question that asks you to select **early** signs of a complication may contain as a distractor an option that lists several **late** signs of the complication.

2. Who is the *client* in the question?

The client is the person who is the focus of the question. The following are examples of who the client may be:

- The person with the health problem
- The person specifically identified in the question as the "client"
- A relative or a neighbor of the person with the health problem
- Another client in the health care setting
- Another staff nurse
- A nursing assistant

It is crucial to identify the client in the question because the answer must relate to the client.

3. What is the *issue* in the question?

The **issue** is the specific problem or subject about which the question is asking. For example, the issue might be:

- A drug (e.g., digoxin, Lasix)
- A problem (e.g., drug addiction, depression)
- A toxic effect of a drug (e.g., nausea, vomiting)
- A behavior (e.g., restlessness, agitation)
- A disorder (e.g., diabetes mellitus, ulcerative colitis)
- A procedure (e.g., glucose tolerance test, cardiac catheterization)

TRUE OR FALSE

4. What is the *type of stem?*

As we have explained, the stem is the part of the question that asks you to solve a problem and select a response. To select the correct option, you need to determine the **type of stem.**

There are two types of stems:

1. **True response stems**
2. **False response stems**

True response stems are questions for which the answer would be an **appropriate** nursing action or an **accurate** explanation. For example, **a true response stem might ask you to identify:**

- An **appropriate** nursing action.
- The **most essential or highest priority** nursing action.
- A **safe** nursing judgment.
- A **therapeutic** nursing response.
- An **accurate** rationale for a nursing action.
- An action or statement by the client **indicating the success** of the nurse's client teaching.
- A **correct explanation** of the difference between two disorders.

In the examples shown below, note the words in **bold** print. These words focus your attention on the "best" or "most correct" option. **Here are some examples of true response stems:**

- Which interpretation of these findings by the nurse is **most** justifiable?
- Which nursing action is **most** important?
- The nurse would demonstrate the **best** judgment by taking which action?
- During the early period, which nursing intervention would be **best**?
- **Initially,** the nurse **should:**
- The nurse understands that the **chief** purpose of the drug is to:
- The nurse should give **immediate** consideration to which symptom?
- The nurse understands that the client is **at risk** for which nursing diagnosis?
- In caring for a male adolescent client, the nurse understands that, as compared to preadolescent boys, **most** adolescent boys **need:**
- Which finding would the nurse identify as **consistent** with the admitting diagnosis?
- The nurse knows that the **similar** characteristic for the client with infectious hepatitis and the client in the first trimester of pregnancy is:
- The nurse **knows that the client understands** how to care for his health problem when the client:

<u>False response stems</u> are those for which the answer would generally be an **inappropriate** nursing action or an **inaccurate** explanation. For example, **a false response stem might ask you to identify:**

- Something the nurse **should not do.**
- The **least essential** or **lowest priority** nursing action.
- A nursing action that **fails to address** the client's problem.
- An **unsafe** nursing judgment.
- A **nontherapeutic** or unhelpful nursing response.
- An **inadequate** or incorrect rationale for a nursing action.
- An **inaccurate** explanation of the difference between two disorders.
- A statement or action by the client indicating a **lack of motivation or understanding** of how to care for a health problem.

In other words, a **false response stem** asks you to select an answer that is **wrong,** or that **has something negative or unimportant about it.**

The following are examples of false response stems. Note the negative word or phrase in **bold** print:

- At this time, which nursing action would be **inappropriate**?
- The nurse knows that which medication would be **contraindicated** for this client?
- The nurse should advise the client to **avoid** taking the medication with:
- The **least important** concern for the nurse to raise with the client at this time is:
- Which nursing action receives the **lowest priority** at this time?
- The nurse would identify that the client **required further instruction** in CPR if the client placed his hands:
- Which nursing action would demonstrate an **unsafe** nursing judgement?
- Which characteristic would the nurse identify as **least likely** to contribute to hypertension?

TECHNIQUE #3

ELIMINATING INCORRECT OPTIONS

After you have identified the four critical elements in a test question, then you can begin to narrow your choices for selecting the correct option. All questions on the NCLEX-RN Exam, and most multiple choice questions that you will find on your nursing course exams, have four options. Of these, three are "distractors" and one is the correct answer.

"Distractors" are incorrect options that are designed to resemble the correct answer. They are intended to "distract" you from answering correctly.

Here is a selection procedure that will help you to eliminate the distractors.

Follow these instructions -- and then see Chapter 4 for some strategies you can use to narrow the choices even further.

❶ First, decide whether the question has a **true response stem** or a **false response stem.**

❷ Then read each of the four options to determine whether it is appropriate/accurate or inappropriate/incorrect (i.e., whether it is a true statement or not.)

If the stem is a *true response stem,* make a decision about each option, as follows:

- **+ This might be the correct answer** because this option is **appropriate**.
- **– This is a distractor** because this option is **inappropriate**.
- **? This is a possibility** because I am **not sure**.

If the stem is a *false response stem,* make a decision about each option, as follows:

- **+ This might be the correct answer** because this option is **inappropriate**.
- **– This is a distractor** because this option is **appropriate**.
- **? This is a possibility** because I am **not sure**.

Sometimes, just applying the test-taking techniques described in this chapter and narrowing your choices for selecting the correct option in the manner described above leads directly to the correct option! When it doesn't, well, keep reading.

HOW TO AVOID MISREADING TEST QUESTIONS

Misreading test questions is a major problem that hinders success on nursing exams. There are many ways in which a question can be misread!

Misreading a test question may happen because you:

1. Incorrectly analyze what the question is really asking.
2. Overlook important words such as "early" or "late," or "unsafe" or "inappropriate."

❸ "Read into" a question information that is not actually given.

❹ Incorrectly interpret a disorder (for example, mistakenly interpreting a complication of diabetes mellitus, such as ketoacidosis, as diabetes mellitus itself).

Here are some test-taking tips to avoid misreading test questions:

❶ Avoid incorrectly analyzing what is being asked:

- **Separate the case scenario and the stem**
- **Identify the client**
- **Identify the issue**
- **Identify the type of stem**

❷ Avoid overlooking important words: **Identify the key words.**

❸ Avoid "reading into" a question:

Try to restate the question in your own words. Then <u>eliminate any option that includes "new" information</u> about the client or the clinical situation that was not given in the case scenario. You should also <u>eliminate any option that requires you to make assumptions about the client</u> involving information not presented in the case scenario.

❹ Avoid misinterpreting disorders:

Review carefully for the exam! Use the method outlined in Chapter Two to review for nursing course exams. For the NCLEX-RN Exam, be sure to follow the plan in Chapter Nine. Focus on any areas in which you have difficulty. Then, use your nursing knowledge and your test-taking techniques when you read each question.

Guidelines to Use when Narrowing the Options

1. By making a decision about each option as you read it, you will save time.
2. You should be able to eliminate at least two options by using this selection procedure.
3. After you have eliminated an option, do not go back to it. Continue to work with the options that are remaining.
4. If you are left with one [+] and one [?], select the [+] as the correct answer. Remember to always go with what you know!
5. Using a selection procedure allows you to make an educated guess when necessary. If you are left with two [+], you have a 50% chance of guessing correctly. If you make a wild guess from all four choices, you have only a 25% chance of guessing correctly.

A Practice Session Focusing on Identifying the Critical Elements and Eliminating Options

As you answer the following questions, remember to ask yourself these questions:

1. What are the key words?
2. Who is the client?
3. What is the issue?
4. What is the stem asking?

Always be sure to determine whether the question has a true response stem or a false stem. When you know the type of stem, then make a decision about each of the options as you read them, by using the selection procedure. After you have answered the question, read the analysis. Note that the **key words** and the **correct answer** are in bold print.

DRILL #1

1. The nurse is admitting a client who is suspected of having diabetes mellitus. If the client does indeed have diabetes mellitus, the nurse would expect to observe:

   A. Shallow, labored respirations.
   B. Increased blood pressure associated with slight periorbital edema.
   C. Periods of altered pulse rate.
   D. Increased urinary output.

ANALYSIS #1

Critical Elements

Key words:	See bold print
Client:	Any client with diabetes mellitus
Issue:	A characteristic of diabetes mellitus
Type of Stem:	True response stem

Eliminate Options

1. The nurse is admitting a client who is suspected of having **diabetes mellitus.** If the client does indeed have diabetes mellitus, the nurse would **expect** to **observe:**

? A. **Shallow, labored** respirations.
Were you tempted by this option? This is a good distractor! It might appear to be a possibility if you thought this was Kussmaul's breathing. However, Kussmaul's breathing is a characteristic of ketoacidosis, which is a complication of diabetes mellitus. This question is about a characteristic of diabetes, not a complication of diabetes. In addition, Kussmaul's breathing is deep and rapid, not shallow and labored.

− B. Increased blood pressure associated with slight periorbital edema.
This is a distractor because this is not a characteristic of diabetes.

? C. Periods of altered pulse rate.
This is a sign of ketoacidosis -- a complication of diabetes -- so you may have thought this was another possibility. This is another distractor, however, because the question specifically asks for a characteristic of diabetes.

\+ D. **Increased urinary output.**
This option is correct. It is the only characteristic of diabetes presented in these four options. Remember the three P's associated with the diagnosis of diabetes mellitus, which are polyuria, polyphagia and polydypsia.

DRILL #2

2. In assessing an adult client with diabetes mellitus, the nurse would identify which finding as unexpected with this diagnosis?

   A. Increased body weight.
   B. Increased urinary output.
   C. Periods of polydypsia.
   D. Alterations in heart rate and rhythm.

ANALYSIS #2

Critical Elements

Key words:	See bold print
Client:	Any adult client
Issue:	A finding that would NOT be observed in an adult with diabetes mellitus
Type of Stem:	False response stem

Eliminate Options

2. In assessing an **adult** client with **diabetes mellitus**, the nurse would identify which finding as **unexpected** with this diagnosis?

➖ A. Increased body weight.
Since the adult diabetic gains weight, this finding would be expected with the diagnosis. The false response stem in this question asks for a finding that would be unexpected. This option is a distractor.

➖ B. Increased urinary output.
Since we are looking for an unexpected finding, this a distractor and not the answer. This is an expected manifestation of adult diabetes.

➖ C. Periods of polydypsia.
This is an expected manifestation of adult diabetes. Since we are looking for an unexpected finding, this is not the answer.

➕ **D. Alterations heart rate and rhythm.**
This question has a false response stem, so the answer is something that the nurse would NOT expect to find in an adult diabetic. Altered heart rate and rhythm are NOT characteristic of diabetes. The other three options are distractors: they list signs and symptoms consistent with the diagnosis of adult diabetes mellitus.

DRILL #3

3. The nurse caring for a client with urolithiasis knows which nursing intervention would be inappropriate?

   A. Forcing fluids.
   B. Straining the urine.
   C. Complete bed rest.
   D. Medication for colic or discomfort.

ANALYSIS #3

Critical Elements

Key words:	See bold print
Client:	Any client with urolithiasis
Issue:	A nursing measure not included in the nursing care of a client with urolithiasis. (To help define urolithiasis, dissect the word: "uro-" is kidney and "lithiasis" is stone)
Type of Stem:	False response stem

Eliminate Options

3. The nurse caring for a client with **urolithiasis** knows which nursing measure would be **inappropriate?**

− A. Forcing fluids.
Nursing care for urolithiasis includes encouraging fluid intake to help flush out the kidney stone. This is a distractor.

− B. Straining the urine.
Nursing care for urolithiasis includes obtaining the stones for analysis, so straining is necessary.

+ **C. Complete bed rest.**
This is the answer to this question with a false response stem. Complete bed rest is inappropriate because the client may ambulate. Ambulation helps the stone to pass through the kidney.

− D. Medication for colic or discomfort.
This is another distractor because nursing care for urolithiasis includes medicating for pain, which can be severe. Remember, the answer is something that is incorrect in the care of a client with a kidney stone.

DRILL #4

4. A client was admitted for a severe episode of gastrointestinal bleeding. Prior to discharge, which statement by the client would indicate to the nurse that the client needs further instruction?

   A. If his arthritis bothers him, he'll take acetaminophen (Tylenol).
   B. He's glad he gave up drinking five years ago.
   C. He can't wait to get home so he can have his morning coffee.
   D. He'll take his cimetidine (Tagamet) before he eats and at bedtime.

ANALYSIS #4

Critical Elements

Key words:	See bold print
Client:	A client with gastrointestinal bleeding
Issue:	A statement by the client that means he does not understand something about his role in caring for himself after an episode of gastrointestinal bleeding
Type of Stem:	False response stem

Eliminate Options

4. A client was admitted for a **severe** episode of **gastrointestinal bleeding.** Prior to discharge, which statement by the client would indicate to the nurse that the client **needs further instruction?**

− A. If his arthritis bothers him, he'll take acetaminophen **(Tylenol).**
Using Tylenol is appropriate for this client (although any aspirin-related drug would be contraindicated because it causes GI bleeding). The stem asks you to identify a statement that indicates that the client does not understand how to care for his health care problem.

− B. He's glad he gave up **drinking** five years ago.
The client's statement indicates that he does understand that caring for his health problem requires avoiding alcohol. Alcohol stimulates the GI tract. Look for a statement indicating that the client does not understand what he should do.

\+ **C. He can't wait to get home so he can have his morning coffee.**
This is the correct answer because such a statement by the client indicates a lack of understanding of how to care for his health problem. Coffee stimulates the GI tract, and it should be avoided. This response

shows that the client needs further education. This is the type of question that can be easily misread!

− D. He'll take his cimetidine **(Tagamet)** before he eats and at bedtime.
The client correctly intends to take the Tagamet before eating and at bedtime. Tagamet is used in the treatment of peptic ulcers to inhibit the secretion of histamine.

DRILL #5

5. The nurse understands that, physiologically, the difference between angina and myocardial infarction is:

A. With angina, arterial perfusion is briefly inadequate. With a myocardial infarction, arterial perfusion is cut off permanently.
B. With angina, the enzymes SGOT, LDH, and CPK are elevated. After a myocardial infarction, they are not elevated.
C. With angina, adrenocorticosteroids are released to reduce the inflammatory reaction. With a myocardial infarction, these hormones are absent.
D. With angina, hypertension and congestive heart failure are absent. With a myocardial infarction, hypertension and congestive heart failure are present.

ANALYSIS #5

Critical Elements

Key words:	See bold print
Client:	Any client with a myocardial infarction or angina
Issue:	The physiological difference between angina and myocardial infarction (Note: This is an example of a question that does not have a case scenario)
Type of Stem:	True response stem

Eliminate Options

5. The nurse understands that, **physiologically**, the **difference** between **angina and myocardial infarction** is:

+ **A. With angina, arterial perfusion is briefly inadequate. With a myocardial infarction, arterial perfusion is cut off permanently.**
This is an accurate comparison, because in a myocardial infarction the blockage of arterial perfusion is permanent and angina involves only temporarily inadequate arterial perfusion. Note: Even though this an-

swer is accurate, you should always read all four options to make sure that this one is the best.

– B. With **angina,** the **enzymes** SGOT, LDH, and CPK are **elevated**. After a myocardial infarction, they are not elevated.
This is an inaccurate comparison; actually, the opposite is true. With an infarction, the enzymes are elevated. Because there is no muscle or tissue damage in angina, the enzymes are not elevated. This is a distractor.

? C. With **angina, adrenocorticosteroids** are **released** to reduce the inflammatory reaction. With a myocardial infarction, these hormones are absent.
This is a good distractor, because it looks like it might be a possible answer. However, this comparison is inaccurate. There is no inflammatory reaction with a myocardial infarction. Did you know that? You probably did! When deciding between two options, always choose what you know for sure.

? D. With **angina, hypertension** and congestive heart failure are **absent**. With a myocardial infarction, hypertension and congestive heart failure are present.
Does this look like another possibility to you? These complications may be associated with either angina or a myocardial infarction, so this comparison is not valid.

All four options in this question are lengthy, but this question is not too difficult. It may take some time to read, however, and you need to read each option carefully!

DRILL #6

6. In contrast to the client with angina, the nurse will observe that the client with a myocardial infarction experiences:

   A. Pain that is relieved by rest and nitroglycerin.
   B. Possible signs of increased cardiac output and hypoxia.
   C. Pain that occurs with increased stress and exercise.
   D. Severe, crushing pain that begins spontaneously.

ANALYSIS #6

Critical Elements

Key words:	See bold print
Client:	Any client with a myocardial infarction
Issue:	A symptom of a myocardial infarction that is not found in angina
Type of Stem:	True response stem (comparison)

Eliminate Options

6. In **contrast** to the client with angina, the nurse will observe that the client with a **myocardial infarction** experiences:

− A. Pain that is relieved by rest and nitroglycerin.
This is a characteristic of angina that is not found in a myocardial infarction. You are looking for just the opposite.

? B. **Possible** signs of **increased** cardiac output and **hypoxia**.
This option may appear to be a possibility. It is true that hypoxia occurs with a myocardial infarction, and the word "possible" may tempt you to choose this option. But there are two symptoms in this option and, for the option to be correct, both symptoms must be associated with a myocardial infarction. Increased cardiac output does not occur with a myocardial infarction; cardiac output is decreased due to the damaged muscle.

− C. Pain that occurs with increased stress and exercise.
These are factors precipitating angina, they are not associated with myocardial infarction. The question is asking for just the opposite.

+ **D. Severe, crushing pain that begins spontaneously.**
Although this type of pain does not occur with all myocardial infarctions, this is most typical of an infarction and not angina. Anginal pain is usually provoked by stress or exercise. Pain associated with a myocardial infarction is usually severe and is not abated by the use of nitroglycerin.

DRILL #7

7. In caring for a 16-year-old client with ulcerative colitis, the nurse understands an important difference between a psychosomatic and a conversion disorder is that in the psychosomatic disorder:

A. The physical symptoms are consciously selected by the person.
B. The physical symptoms are relieved when the mental conflict is resolved.
C. The physical symptoms may be fatal if left untreated.
D. The person characteristically has an attitude of indifference toward the physical symptoms.

ANALYSIS #7

Critical Elements

Key words:	See bold print
Client:	A 16-year-old with ulcerative colitis
Issue:	An aspect of a psychosomatic disorder that does not apply to a conversion disorder.
Type of Stem:	True response stem (comparison)

Eliminate Options

7. In caring for a 16-year-old client with **ulcerative colitis,** the nurse understands an **important difference** between a psychosomatic and a **conversion** disorder is that **in the psychosomatic disorder:**

− A. The physical symptoms are **consciously** selected by the person.
The physical symptoms are not consciously selected in either illness. Look for an accurate statement about a psychosomatic disorder that is not true for a conversion disorder.

? B. The physical symptoms **are relieved** when the mental conflict is resolved.
This a good distractor, because it might be a possibility. However, this is true of both illnesses. In both psychosomatic and conversion disorders, the symptoms decrease as the mental conflict is relieved. The issue of the question is the difference between these two illnesses.

\+ C. **The physical symptoms may be fatal if left untreated.**
This is the major difference between these two illnesses. The client with a psychophysiological (psychosomatic) disorder may die from their illness if there is no medical intervention. The client with a conversion disorder (a hypochondriac) will not die from their physical symptoms. Note that this question could have been asked without any reference to an actual client. The drafter of this question tossed in a big clue by providing a client with ulcerative colitis, which can be life-threatening if it is not treated. That is another reason to identify key words: to take advantage of those free hints!

− D. The person characteristically has an attitude of **indifference** toward the physical symptoms.
This is not an accurate statement about a client with ulcerative colitis, who is most likely very concerned about their medical problem because it is life-threatening. This is a characteristic of a conversion disorder.

In this chapter, two important test-taking strategies were introduced. In addition to these strategies, some important points when answering test questions are listed on the following page.

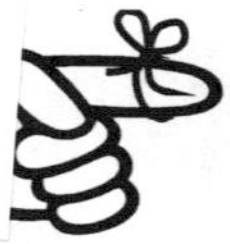

Points to Remember

❶ Answer questions as if the situation were ideal and the nurse had all the time and resources needed. The only client you need to be concerned about is the one in the question!

❷ Be sure to identify the false response stems which ask you to select an inappropriate nursing action or an inaccurate rationale or comparison. These questions are easy to <u>misread.</u>

❸ Lengthy questions are not always difficult!

❹ Certain words like "possible," "usually," or "may," will often make a statement true and may make that option a "possible ?" answer. On the other hand, absolute terms like "always" or "never" tend to make a statement incorrect.

❺ Make sure to read all of the options -- and <u>then</u> select the best!

Chapter 4

~~1. Option 1~~
? 2. Option 2
~~3. Option 3~~
? 4. Option 4

How Do I Choose Between the Two Best Options?

In most nursing exam questions, often it is easy to eliminate two distractors. The two remaining options, however, often appear equally correct. For example, of four possible nursing interventions, two may be inappropriate and easily ruled out, but both of the remaining two may appear quite appropriate. Or you may have difficulty deciding between two possible options that appear to be very close in meaning. So how do you decide between two possible options?

You receive credit only for identifying the correct answer. You do not receive any credit for identifying the best distractors! Although two choices may seem equally good, **one is always better and more correct.**

The following test-taking strategies will help you to choose between the two best options. If you are unable to choose the answer using your nursing knowledge, you should apply the strategies rather than just guess at the answer. In this chapter, **you will learn three strategies that will help you master the skill of eliminating incorrect options and choosing the correct answer.**

NOTE➤

The test-taking strategies presented in this chapter will require that you understand the test-taking terminology and techniques presented in Chapter Three. If you have not yet read Chapter Three, do so before proceeding with Chapter Four.

STRATEGY #1

THE GLOBAL RESPONSE

When more than one option appears to be correct, **look for a global response.**

A global response is one that is a general statement and may include the ideas of other options within it.

This option is often the correct answer when two or three more specific options appear equally correct.

A Practice Session Focusing on Looking for the Global Response

Read and answer the following questions, looking for an option that is more global than the others. First, review the questions by identifying the four critical elements. Then narrow your choices, and look for the option that includes a global response. After you have answered the question, read the Analysis. Note that the **key words** and the **answer** are shown in bold print.

DRILL #1

1. The nurse understands that the overall aim of therapy for a client with cerebral palsy is to:

   A. Improve muscle control and coordination.
   B. Correct the underlying cause of the disease.
   C. Prevent contractures and emotional disturbances.
   D. Maximize the client's assets and minimize his limitations.

ANALYSIS #1

Critical Elements

Key words:	See bold print
Client:	Any client with cerebral palsy
Issue:	The overall aim of therapy for cerebral palsy
Type of Stem:	True response stem

Eliminate Options

1. The nurse understands that the **overall aim** of therapy for a client with **cerebral palsy** is to:

? A. Improve muscle control and coordination.
This is an appropriate goal of therapy in cerebral palsy and a possibility. Since cerebral palsy causes spasticity of the muscles and gross and fine motor incoordination, muscle training is needed. By reading on, however, you can see that this is too specific and not global enough to be the best statement of the overall aim of therapy. Always make sure you read all the options before selecting the best one!

– B. Correct the underlying cause of the disease.
This is an inappropriate goal, since cerebral palsy is a nonprogressive motor disorder that stems from permanent damage to the motor centers and pathways in the brain. Correcting the underlying cause is not medically possible.

? C. Prevent contractures and emotional disturbances.
This is a possibility and another good distractor, because it is an appropriate goal in cerebral palsy. This is one goal of therapy, since communication and self-help deficits and spasticity cause contractures and emotional problems. Like option A, this is another specific goal.

+ **D. Maximize the client's assets and minimize his limitations.**
This is the best option because it is the most complete or global answer to the question. Note that this option encompasses the ideas of options A and C.

DRILL #2

2. The nurse assigned to care for a child with cerebral palsy should obtain information concerning the child's abilities, limitations, interests and habits, because the aim of therapy is to:

A. Assess the child's assets and potentialities and capitalize on these in the rehabilitative process, while overlooking limitations.
B. Reverse abnormal functioning and restore brain damage through rehabilitation.
C. Provide a therapeutic program that avoids subjecting the child to frustrating experiences that decrease his achievement.
D. Develop an individualized therapeutic program that utilizes the child's assets and abilities, and provides experiences that permit him to achieve success as well as help him to cope with frustration and failure.

ANALYSIS #2

Critical Elements

Key words:	See bold print
Client:	A child with cerebral palsy
Issue:	The aim of therapy for cerebral palsy
Type of Stem:	True response stem

Eliminate Options

2. The nurse who is assigned to care for a child with **cerebral palsy** should obtain information concerning his abilities, limitations, interests and habits because the **aim** of **therapy** is to:

− A. Assess the child's assets and potentialities and capitalize on these in the rehabilitative process while **overlooking** his limitations.
Part of the goal statement is appropriate, but part of it is inappropriate, which makes the whole option incorrect. It is never an aim of therapy to overlook the client's limitations.

− B. Reverse abnormal functioning and **restore** brain damage through rehabilitation.
This is definitely an inappropriate goal, since cerebral palsy results in permanent malfunction of the motor centers. Brain damage cannot be reversed or restored.

− C. Provide a therapeutic program that **avoids** subjecting the child to frustrating experiences that decrease his achievement.
This goal is inappropriate because of the word "avoid." The aim of therapy is not to avoid a frustrating experience. This would be also be unrealistic.

+ **D. Develop an individualized therapeutic program that utilizes the child's assets and abilities and provides experiences that permit him to achieve success as well as help to cope with frustration and failure.**
This is an appropriate goal for cerebral palsy. This is also a global option and the best goal statement, since it includes recognizing the client's assets and helping the child to cope with frustrations and failures due to his limitations. This is a lengthy option that is comprehensive.

DRILL #3

3. A client says, "I am having a real problem getting pregnant. What could be wrong?" Which ideas should be incorporated into the nurse's response?

   A. Infertility is often caused by congenital anomalies of the reproductive organs.
   B. Infertility is sometimes precipitated by the use of over-the-counter drugs.
   C. Infertility is frequently caused by multiple factors rather than a single factor.
   D. Emotional problems, including stress, can cause a decrease in fertility.

ANALYSIS #3

Critical Elements

Key words:	See bold print
Client:	A child with cerebral palsy
Issue:	The aim of therapy for cerebral palsy
Type of Stem:	True response stem

Eliminate Options

3. A client says, "I am having a **real problem getting pregnant.** What could be wrong?" Which ideas should be incorporated into the **nurse's response**?

? A. Infertility is **often** caused by congenital anomalies of the reproductive organs.
This is a possible answer because the word "often" makes the information it contains true. However, this is just one possible factor, and the case scenario does not present much information about the client. Look for a more global response.

? B. Infertility is **sometimes** precipitated by the use of over-the-counter drugs.
This is another possible answer because of the word "sometimes," but like option A this is just one possible cause.

\+ **C. Infertility is frequently caused by multiple factors rather than a single factor.**
This is the correct option because it is the most global. The "multiple factors" may include congenital anomalies, over-the-counter drugs, and emotional difficulties. When two options contain correct information but are very specific, with no reason to prefer one to the other, look for an option that is more global. This option is the most comprehensive.

? D. Emotional difficulties, including stress, can cause a decrease in fertility. *This is another possibility because the information it contains is correct. However, this option is also too specific.*

STRATEGY #2

SIMILAR DISTRACTORS

If you don't know the answer, your second strategy is to look for similar distractors. Remember that there is only one best option. If two options essentially say the same thing or include the same idea, then neither of these options can be the answer. The answer has to be the option that is different. This is a difficult strategy to understand. The following illustrative questions will help to clarify this strategy. This is an excellent strategy to learn and use.

A Practice Session Focusing on Looking for Similar Distractors

Read and answer the following questions, eliminating the options that are similar. First, read the questions, identify the four critical elements and narrow your choices. Then practice using the similar distractor strategy by looking for the option that is different. After you have answered the question, read the Analysis. The **key words** and the **answer** are in bold print.

DRILL #4

4. To monitor a client for the most common complication arising from the administration of total parenteral nutrition, the nurse should:

A. Weigh the client at the same time each day using the same scale.
B. Keep accurate records of total intake and total output.
C. Determine the increase or decrease in body weight each day.
D. Take the client's temperature at least every four hours.

ANALYSIS #4

Critical Elements

Key words:	See bold print
Client:	Any client receiving total parenteral nutrition
Issue:	Monitoring for the most common complication from TPN
Type of Stem:	True response stem

Eliminate Options

4. To **monitor** a client for the **most common complication** arising from the administration of **total parenteral nutrition,** the nurse should:

? A. Weigh the client at the same time each day using the same scale.
This is a good distractor, since it is a possibility. This nursing action is needed to assess adequate nutrition. The purpose of TPN is to provide adequate nutrition. The flow rate must be regulated. If the rate is too fast, hypermolar diuresis occurs. If the rate is too slow, inadequate nutrition occurs. By weighing the client daily using the same scale, the nurse is assessing adequate nutrition. Since you have identified the issue, however, you know that you are looking for a common complication of TPN. Remember to read all the options before making your decision.

? B. Keep accurate records of total intake and total output.
This is another appropriate nursing action and a possible option. Again, the reason to assess intake and output is to assess for adequate nutrition. This option is very similar to option A. Since both refer to the same idea, however, neither of these options can be the correct answer. Look for the option that is different.

? C. Determine the increase or decrease in body weight each day.
This option is similar to Options A and B and yet another possible option. All of the options so far are concerned with monitoring adequate nutrition. Again, since all three options refer to the same idea, neither of them can be the correct answer. The answer then has to be D.

\+ **D. Take the client's temperature at least every four hours.**
This is the only option that addresses the issue in the question, which is monitoring for a common complication of TPN. Catheter-related infections are the most common complication of TPN. Options A, B, and C all address weight and are so similar that there is no reason to prefer one of them over the others. Option D is the "different" option and the correct answer. Using the strategy of eliminating similar distractors can improve your understanding of "test question logic" and increase your score!

DRILL #5

5. A newly diagnosed adult diabetic is doing a return demonstration of the proper technique for insulin injection. He draws up the correct dose of insulin using the proper technique, but when he is ready to inject the needle, he hesitates and says, "I'm not sure I can do this." Which response by the nurse would be best initially?

A. "I'll show you again how to inject the needle."
B. "I'll inject the needle for you this time."
C. "You're doing fine so far. Give it a try."
D. "Why are you so nervous? Do you need help?"

ANALYSIS #5

Critical Elements

Key words:	See bold print
Client:	A newly diagnosed adult diabetic
Issue:	The nurse's initial response to an unsure client doing a return demonstration
Type of Stem:	True response stem

Eliminate Options

5. A **newly** diagnosed adult diabetic, is doing a **return demonstration** of the proper technique for insulin injection. He draws up the correct dose of insulin using the proper technique, but when he is ready to inject the needle, he hesitates and says, "I'm **not sure** I can do this." Which response by the nurse would be best **initially?**

? A. "I'll show you again how to inject the needle."
This response is a possibility, since this nursing action may sometimes be appropriate in client teaching. This case scenario states that the client is using the proper technique in the return demonstration. This response is not the best one because it focuses on the nurse doing the procedure rather than on the client doing the procedure. Remember, the purpose of nursing is to help the client maintain an optimal level of functioning.

? B. "I'll inject the needle for you this time."
This is also a possibility, but this is similar to option B in that the nurse does the procedure.

\+ **C. "You're doing fine so far. Give it a try."**
This is the correct answer because it focuses on the client doing the procedure himself. The nurse encourages the client to do the procedure for himself. This answer is client-centered.

− D. "Why are you so nervous? Do you need help?"
"Why" responses are always incorrect. This response blocks communication by making the client feel defensive. This response is not therapeu-

tic because it focuses on the client's nervousness and need for help. Being nervous and unsure is an appropriate feeling for this newly diagnosed adult diabetic. The nurse's response should enhance the client's feelings of competency.

DRILL #6

6. In providing care to a client with COPD, the primary nursing consideration is to:

   A. Not overtire the client.
   B. Plan adequate rest periods throughout the day.
   C. Give only low flow oxygen.
   D. Allow the client to move at his own pace.

ANALYSIS #6

Critical Elements

Key words:	See bold print
Client:	Any client with COPD
Issue:	A primary nursing consideration for a client with COPD
Type of Stem:	True response stem

Eliminate Options

6. In providing care to a client with **COPD,** the **primary** nursing consideration is to:

? A. Not overtire the client.
This is a possible answer. A client with COPD needs to avoid activities that produce excessive shortage of breath to preserve existing pulmonary function. You need to continue reading and see if you think that this is the best option.

? B. To plan adequate rest periods throughout the day.
This is another possible answer, but it is similar to option A. Both refer to rest as the primary nursing consideration in caring for a client with COPD. Since both A and B present the same idea, neither can be the answer.

\+ C. **To give only low flow oxygen.**
This is the correct answer in this question that asks you to select an option reflecting a nursing priority. After reading all the options, you

will find that this is the best one. With the diagnosis of COPD, it is important not to remove the hypoxic drive by providing too much oxygen, which can lead to hypoventilation and respiratory insufficiency. This is the only option that refers to the COPD client's special need to maintain low levels of oxygen.

? D. To allow the client to move at his own pace.
This is a possible answer because it would be appropriate. Using the similar distractor test-taking strategy, however, you can eliminate this option because, like options A and B, it is based on the idea of rest.

STRATEGY #3

SIMILAR WORDS

If you don't know the answer, look first for a global response option and try to eliminate similar distractors. If you still cannot choose between the two best options, look for a similar word or phrase used in the stem of the question and in one of the options. If you find a word, feeling, or behavior used in the stem or the case scenario that is repeated in one of the options, that option may be the correct answer. Although looking for similar words is not as reliable as the first two strategies in this chapter, it is helpful when you can't decide on the best answer and the other two strategies cannot be used.

A Practice Session Focusing on Looking for Similar Words

As you read and answer the following questions, look for an answer that has a similar word or phrase in the stem of the question and in one of the options. First, review the questions by identifying the four critical elements. Then narrow your choices while looking for the option that includes a similar word. After you have answered the question, read the Analysis. The key words and the answers are in bold print.

DRILL #7

7. In caring for a client immediately following a cardiac catheterization procedure, which nursing action is appropriate?

A. Applying warm compresses to the puncture site.
B. Assisting with passive range of motion exercises.
C. Monitoring the client for cardiac arrhythmias.
D. Assisting the client into high Fowler's position.

ANALYSIS #7

Critical Elements

Key words: See bold print
Client: Any client following a cardiac catheterization
Issue: A vital nursing action immediately after a cardiac catheterization
Type of Stem: True response stem

Eliminate Options

7. In caring for a client **immediately** following a **cardiac catheterization** procedure, which nursing action is **appropriate?**

− A. Apply warm compresses to the puncture site.
This action is unsafe! Because bleeding and hematoma are major complications in the post procedure period, heat is never applied.

− B. Assist with passive range of motion exercises.
This action is also unsafe. Because of the complication of bleeding, movement is limited in the involved extremity.

+ C. **Monitor the client for cardiac arrhythmias.**
Irregularities in the heart rate are a vital concern in the post procedure period. Until the vital signs are stable, the client needs to be closely assessed for arrhythmias. This is the correct answer. Note that the word "cardiac" is also used in the stem.

− D. Assist the client into high Fowler's position.
This is unsafe. This position could obstruct arterial blood flow and lead to formation of a thrombus. The extremity used for the site must be properly aligned and immobilized immediately after the procedure.

DRILL #8

8. A 22-year-old client sustained a fracture of the tibia and fibula while playing football. In providing care for this client, who has a newly applied long leg cast, which consideration is vital?

A. Elevation of the leg in the cast on a pillow will minimize edema.
B. Healing of a fractured bone requires an extended period of time.
C. A long period of immobility may lead to atrophy of the muscle.
D. Analgesics may be needed for pain associated with the fracture.

ANALYSIS #8

Critical Elements

Key words:	See bold print
Client:	A 22-year-old client with a fractured tibia and fibula
Issue:	A vital consideration when caring for a client with a newly applied cast
Type of Stem:	True response stem

Eliminate Options

8. A 22-year-old client has sustained a fracture of the tibia and fibula while playing football. In providing nursing care for this client, who has a **newly applied long leg cast,** which consideration is **vital?**

\+ A. **Elevation of the leg in the cast on a pillow will minimize edema.**
When caring for a client with a newly applied cast, it is important to keep the affected extremity above the level of the heart to reduce swelling. Swelling causes vasoconstriction. Note that the words "leg" and "cast" are repeated in this option.

? B. Healing of a fractured bone requires an extended period of time.
This option might be a possible answer, since this statement correctly states the pathophysiology of a fracture. The issue in the question, however, is a vital action when caring for a client with a newly applied cast. This option does not address the issue of the question.

? C. A long period of immobility may lead to atrophy of the muscle.
Like option B, this option contains correct information, so it appears to be a possible choice, but it, too, relates to the pathophysiology issue. The focus of the answer has to be a vital nursing consideration.

\+ D. Analgesics may be needed for pain associated with the fracture.
This nursing action is necessary in caring for a fracture. However, the issue is nursing care associated with a newly applied cast, not a fracture, and this is not the most vital consideration. Note that in this question there were two very good answers, only one of which was correct because it alone answered the question actually being asked. It is not just coincidence that the one correct answer repeated the words "leg" and "cast."

DRILL #9

9. Four weeks after a fracture of the tibia and fibula, the nurse notes decreased breath sounds in the lower lobes of both lungs. What is the nurse's best explanation of this change in breath sounds?

   A. The client did not take deep breaths while the nurse examined the lower lobes.
   B. Because of improper positioning, the client has developed pulmonary edema.
   C. Atelectasis caused by immobility resulted in the decreased breath sounds.
   D. The client's resistance is down, and he has caught a cold from someone else.

ANALYSIS #9

Critical Elements

Key words:	See bold print
Client:	Any client with decreased breath sounds
Issue:	Possible rationale for decreased breath sounds four weeks after a fracture
Type of Stem:	True response stem

Eliminate Options

9. **Four weeks** after a fracture of the tibia and fibula the nurse notes **decreased breath sounds** in the lower lobes of both lungs. What is the nurse's best explanation of this change in **breath sounds?**

? A. The client did not take deep breaths while the nurse examined the lower lobes.
This might seem to be a possible explanation, but this option introduces new information not found in the case scenario. There is no information that the client did not take deep breaths. If you chose this option, you "read into" the question.

– B. Because of improper positioning, the client has developed pulmonary edema.
Pulmonary edema is usually not a complication caused by immobility from a fracture and would not be the reason for the decreased breath sounds. Pulmonary edema is a complication of heart failure. This option also "read into" the question by adding the improper positioning rationale.

+ C. **Atelectasis caused by immobility resulted in the decreased breath sounds.**
Immobility causes atelectasis, which results in decreased breath sounds. This is the most plausible reason for the decreased breath sounds. This is a fairly difficult question. Note that the words "breath sounds" used in the stem are repeated in this option.

− D. The client's resistance is down and he has caught a cold from someone else.
Since there is <u>*no information*</u> *in the case scenario about the client having a cold, this is not the answer. Be careful not to "read into" the question.*

Here are some important points to remember from this chapter:

Points to Remember

❶ If you are unable to answer using your nursing knowledge alone, then apply strategies!

❷ When more than one option appears correct, lokk for:

- A global response, or
- Similar distractors that you can eliminate, or
- A similar word or phrase used in both the case scenario (or stem) and one of the options

Chapter 5

Learning to Answer Communication Questions

Communication is an essential skill in the practice of nursing. The goal of nursing is to help the client attain and maintain an optimal level of functioning. Communication skills are needed to achieve this nursing goal. Since the NCLEX-RN Exam measures your ability to practice safely, communication skills are an integral part of the exam.

If you cannot communicate therapeutically, it is difficult to practice safely.

For this reason, your exams in your nursing courses may also include many communication questions.

Communication skills are recognized as vital at all levels of nursing practice. Today there are communication test questions on every type of certification exam in nursing practice, including the specialty levels. Learning how to answer communication questions will enhance your score on the NCLEX-RN Exam and on other nursing exams.

Students frequently report that there are a great number of questions that refer to the psychiatric clinical setting on NCLEX-RN Exam. Many of these "psych" questions are actually communication questions. According to the NCLEX-RN Exam Test Plan (see Chapter Nine), the communication thread is a major component of the exam.

NOTE➤

The test-taking strategies presented in this chapter will require that you understand the test-taking terminology and techniques presented in Chapters Three and Four. If you have not yet read those chapters, do so before proceeding with Chapter Five. You also should read the Introduction.

Identifying the Client in a Communication Question

You want to start with the test-taking techniques that you learned in Chapter Three. When you identify the critical elements, however, two elements require particular attention. First, you must take care when you identify **the client in the question.** This is not always obvious to the unskilled test-taker, because **the client is not necessarily the person identified with the health problem.**

The client in the question is the person to whom the nurse must respond -- and this is almost always someone in the case scenario who has asked the nurse something, or perhaps someone who has done something that affects the nurse. Depending upon the question's case scenario and the stem of the question, the client may be a relative, another client, or even another nurse. As in other types of questions, you need to determine exactly what the question is **asking** before you can answer it.

Identifying the Issue

When you identify the issue in the question be prepared for some twists based on who is the actual client in the question. The issue must relate to the client in the question, and the nurse's response must address the client's issue. Thus, you may get detailed clinical information about a critically ill client whose wife asks the nurse about visiting hours. You must be able to spot the fact that the wife is the client in the question and that the issue then will pertain to her.

Communication Tools and Blocks

Once you have identified the critical elements, particularly the client in the question, the issue, and the type of stem, you need to select your answer. To do this, you need to apply your knowledge of therapeutic communication. The following guidelines summarize the **tools** and **blocks** to therapeutic communication.

Communication tools are mechanisms that **enhance** therapeutic communication. The blocks are responses that **interfere** with communication. Examples of the therapeutic communication tools are shown in the following table.

Therapeutic Communication Tools

Tools	Examples of statements
Being silent	Sitting quietly
Offering self	"Let me sit with you."
Showing empathy	"You are upset."
Focusing	"You say that..."
Restatement	"You feel anxious?"
Validation/clarification	"What you are saying is...?"
Giving information	"Your room is 423."
Dealing with the here and now	"At this time, the problem is..."

The nurse must be in a therapeutic role. When you answer communication questions, remember that **only options that use therapeutic communication <u>tools</u> can be correct answers (if the question has a true response stem).**

Examples of blocks to communication are shown in the table below. Keep in mind that **blocks are the distractors and tools are the answers.** After reviewing the tools and blocks, apply these concepts to the questions in the practice session.

Communication Blocks

Blocks	Examples of statements
Giving advice	"If I were you, I would..."
Showing approval/disapproval	"You did the right thing."
Using cliche and false reassurance	"Don't worry. It will be all right."
Requesting an explanation	"Why did you do that?"
Devaluing client feelings	"Don't be concerned. It's not a problem?"
Being defensive	"Every nurse on this unit is exceptional."
Focusing on inappropriate issues or persons	"Have I said something wrong?"
Placing the client's issues on "hold"	"Talk to your doctor about that."

NOTE➤

A final point to note in answering communication questions is that the nurse must put special emphasis on recognizing and responding to the client's feelings.

Q&A

A Practice Session Focusing on Learning to Answer Communication Questions

Read and answer the following questions. When selecting the best response by the nurse, look for the response that enhances communication. Remember to identify the critical elements, especially the client in the question and the issue.

When you have identified the type of stem, narrow your choices, looking for responses by the nurse that use communication tools and responses that address the client's feelings. Remember to apply the three test-taking strategies from Chapter Four, too; these strategies are also extremely useful in communication questions. After you have answered the question, read the analysis. **Key words** and the **correct answers** are in bold print.

DRILL #1

1. A 78-year-old client is admitted to the hospital for an exploratory laparotomy. The client's daughter says to the nurse, "I wish I could stay with my father, but I need to go home to see how my children are doing. I really hate to leave my father alone at this time." The best nursing response is:

   A. "Your father needs opportunities to be independent. This will help him become self-sufficient."
   B. "Your father is capable of taking care of himself. Try allowing him more independence."
   C. "Stress is not good for your father at this time. Perhaps you could call your children."
   D. "You are feeling concern for both your father and your children. Let me know when you are leaving, and I'll stay with him."

ANALYSIS #1

Critical Elements

Key words:	See bold print
Client:	The daughter
Issue:	A response to the daughter's concerns about needing to leave her father alone
Type of Stem:	True response stem (therapeutic communication)

Eliminate Options

1. A **78-year-old** client is admitted to the hospital for an **exploratory laparotomy**. The **client's daughter says** to the nurse, **"I wish I could stay** with my father, **but I need to go home** to see how my children are doing. **I really hate to leave my father alone** at this time." The **best** nursing response is:

− A. "Your father needs opportunities to be independent. This will help him become self-sufficient."
This is a block to communication because it is giving advice. The daughter is the client in this question, and this response fails to address the client's issue, which is her immediate concern about leaving her father.

− B. "Your father is capable of taking care of himself. Try allowing him more independence."
This is also the communication block of giving advice. Like option A, this response does not address the daughter's immediate concern about leaving her father.

− C. "Stress is not good for your father at this time. Perhaps you could call your children."
Like options A and B, this is giving advice and another block to communication. The answer has to be D.

\+ **D. "You are feeling concern for both your father and your children. Let me know when you are leaving, and I'll stay with him."**
This response uses the tools of empathy and offering self. This empathetic response focuses on the client's concerns of the moment, of being both a mother and a daughter, which she has shared with the nurse. The nurse uses the tool of offering self by offering to stay with the father.

DRILL #2

2. An elderly male client who is hospitalized for an exploratory laparotomy says to the nurse, "Do you think that the doctor can fix whatever is wrong with me?" Which response by the nurse would be best initially?

A. "That question can only be answered after your surgery."
B. "People your age frequently have problems that can be corrected by surgery."
C. "You need to get more information from your doctor."
D. "You must be worried about what the doctor might find."

ANALYSIS #2

Critical Elements

Key words:	See bold print
Client:	An elderly client hospitalized for an exploratory laparotomy
Issue:	The client's concerns about possible findings
Type of Stem:	True response stem (therapeutic communication)

Eliminate Options

2. An **elderly** client who is hospitalized for an **exploratory laparotomy says** to the nurse, "Do you think that the doctor can fix **whatever is wrong with me?"** Which response by the nurse would be best **initially**?

− A. "That question can only be answered after your surgery."
The question asks which response is best initially. This is a block that places the client's feelings on hold. This response might be suitable for a later time, after the nurse has addressed the client's feelings.

− B. "People your age frequently have problems that can be corrected by surgery."
This statement may or may not be true; however, the case scenario does not include any information to indicate that the client's suspected health problem is related to age. This response cannot be the answer because it blocks communication by giving false reassurance. It also refers to inappropriate persons ("people your age") and, directly related to that block, it fails to address the client's feelings.

− C. "You need to get more information from your doctor."
In this response the nurse fails to address the client's concerns and feelings. This response is a block that puts the client's feelings on hold. This response is not therapeutic.

+ **D. "You must be worried about what the doctor might find."**
This is the correct answer, because this response uses two therapeutic communication tools. One is empathy, which is shown by focusing on the client's feelings. The second tool is restatement, a tool that helps the client clarify his feelings. Communication theory identifies that the nurse should address the client's feelings, so the "initial response" often will be one that focuses on the client's feelings. After the client's feelings are addressed, information can be more productively communicated.

DRILL #3

3. A 20-day-old infant is recovering from surgery for pyloric stenosis. The mother asks the nurse, "Now that my son has had this surgery, is it likely that pyloric stenosis will cause trouble later?" Which is the most appropriate nursing response?

   A. "Why don't you talk to the doctor about your uncertainties regarding your son's future?"
   B. "He might develop obstructive symptoms later. If so, take him immediately to an emergency room."
   C. "He will not have symptoms again in childhood, but may have digestive difficulties in his adult life."
   D. "Recurrence of the obstruction or repetition of the surgical procedure would be unlikely."

ANALYSIS #3

Critical Elements

Key words:	See bold print
Client:	The mother
Issue:	Mother's concern regarding prognosis for son with pyloric stenosis
Type of Stem:	True response stem (therapeutic communication)

Eliminate Options

3. A 20-day-old infant is recovering from surgery for **pyloric stenosis**. The **mother** asks the nurse, "Now that my son has had this surgery, is it likely that pyloric stenosis will cause **trouble later?"** Which is the most **appropriate** nursing response?

[–] A. "Why don't you talk to the doctor about your uncertainties regarding your son's future?"
This responses uses the <u>*block*</u> *of placing the client's concerns on hold. The nurse needs to address the issue here and now.*

[?] B. "He might develop obstructive symptoms later. If so, take him **immediately** to an emergency room."
This is a <u>*possibility*</u>*. It is true that pyloric stenosis may recur, but this option does not fully answer her question and will increase her fear. Remember, if part of the option is correct and part is incorrect, it makes the whole option wrong.*

− C. "He **will not** have symptoms again in childhood, but may have digestive difficulties in his adult life."
This is too absolute a statement and it is therefore <u>inaccurate</u> information. The nurse cannot say with absolute certainty that the baby will not have symptoms again in childhood. Recurrence is remotely possible.

\+ **D. "Recurrence of the obstruction or repetition of the surgical procedure would be unlikely."**
This option uses the <u>tool</u> of giving information, responding to the mother's concern by providing information that is accurate. A better response might also address the mother's feelings, but no such response is offered with this question. Of all the options, this is the best. You may not like any of the choices, but you cannot skip questions and so need to select the best option.

DRILL #4

4. A few days after being admitted following a drinking binge, a chronic alcoholic client becomes increasingly agitated and tells the staff that red ants are walking all over the floor and walls. The nurse enters the room and finds the client shouting in a terrified voice, "Get those ants out of my room." Which nursing response is most therapeutic at this time?

A. "Tell me more about the ants that you see in your room."
B. "I'm sure that the ants you see will not harm you."
C. "I don't see any ants, but you seem very frightened."
D. "I do not see anything. This is part of your illness."

ANALYSIS #4

Critical Elements

Key words:	See bold print
Client:	A chronic alcoholic client who is hallucinating
Issue:	Response to a hallucinating alcoholic client who is terrified
Type of Stem:	True response stem (therapeutic communication)

Eliminate Options

4. A few days after being admitted following a drinking binge, a chronic alcoholic client becomes increasingly **agitated** and tells the staff that **red ants** are walking all over the floor and walls. The nurse enters the room and finds the client shouting in a **terrified** voice, "Get those ants out of my room." Which of the following comments would be **most appropriate** at this time?

− A. "Tell me more about the ants you see in your room."
This is not therapeutic because it blocks communication by focusing on the ants or the mechanics of the hallucination, rather than on the client's feelings.

− B. "I'm sure that the ants you see will not harm you."
This response uses the block of false reassurance -- at least the client will perceive it this way! This response also is nontherapeutic because in dealing with hallucinations it is inappropriate to reinforce the hallucination. In this case scenario, the nurse needs to reinforce reality and address the client's feelings.

\+ **C. "I don't see any ants, but you seem very frightened."**
This response presents reality in an appropriate manner and uses the communication tool of empathy to address the client's feelings. By saying, "you seem frightened," the nurse acknowledges the client's feelings that have been communicated in his terrified voice. Note that the test-taking strategy of observing a similar word in the case scenario and one of the options can be successfully used here: the words "frightened" and "terrified" are similar.

? D. "I do not see anything. This is part of your illness."
This might be a possibility, since this option does present reality; however, this response does not address the client's feelings. Option C is better because it uses the tool of empathy.

DRILL #5

5. After one week of hospitalization, a chronic alcoholic client's son visits and says to the nurse, "I would do anything if my dad would only stop drinking." What would be the initial goal of the nurse's response?

A. To have the son join a support group like Al-Anon.
B. To reinforce that the family is very supportive of his father.
C. To help the son understand that his father needs to take responsibility for his disease.
D. To help him explain the problem as he sees it.

ANALYSIS #5

Critical Elements

Key words:	See bold print
Client:	The son
Issue:	An alcoholic's son's concerns about his father
Type of Stem:	True response stem (therapeutic communication)

Eliminate Options

5. After one week of hospitalization, a chronic alcoholic's **son** visits and says to the nurse, "I would do anything if my dad would only stop drinking." What would be the **initial goal** of the nurse's response?

? A. Have him join a support group like Al-Anon.
This goal is appropriate and is a possibility. However, this question asks for the initial goal regarding the son's present concerns. This option fails to address the son's concern and blocks communication by advising.

− B. Reinforce that the family is very supportive of his father.
This is another block because it gives false reassurance and does not focus on the son's concerns. This response could also be interpreted as the nurse giving approval, which is nontherapeutic.

? C. Help him understand that his father needs to take responsibility for his disease.
This is a possibility, however, this question asks about the initial goal. This might be a goal for later.

+ **D. Help him explain the problem as he sees it.**
This response uses the tool of clarification. In order for the son to resolve his problem, the problem needs to be defined. This response helps him clarify his problem. This also reflects the first step of the nursing process, which is assessment. By helping the son to clarify the problem, the nurse is gathering additional information about the son's concern. Before a nursing diagnosis can be made, the nurse must identify and clarify the problem. In Chapter Six you will learn even more about using the nursing process to answer test questions.

DRILL #6

6. During a lengthy conversation with the nurse about his long history of alcoholism, a client becomes tense and uncomfortable. He begins biting his lip and tightly clutching his hands. At this time, which of the following remarks by the nurse would be the most appropriate?

A. "What did I say to make you feel uncomfortable?"
B. "Drinking for a long period of time can make anyone feel uncomfortable."
C. "At what point did you begin to feel uncomfortable?"
D. "You need to talk about your long drinking history if you are to recover from your illness."

ANALYSIS #6

Critical Elements

Key words:	See bold print
Client:	A chronic alcoholic
Issue:	The client's tenseness when talking about his long history of drinking
Type of Stem:	True response stem (therapeutic communication)

Eliminate Options

6. During a lengthy conversation with the nurse about his long history of alcoholism, the client becomes **tense and uncomfortable.** He begins biting his lip and tightly clutching his hands. **At this time,** which of the following remarks would be the **most appropriate**?

? A. "What did I say to make you feel uncomfortable?"
This might appear to be a possibility and it is a good distractor. This option actually blocks communication because it focuses on an inappropriate person (the nurse)rather than on the client. The nurse is accepting responsibility for the client's feelings. A therapeutic response focuses on the client rather than on the nurse.

– B. "Drinking for a long period of time can make anyone feel uncomfortable."
This response is a block that devalues the client's feelings. It's like saying, "We all get depressed."

\+ C. **"At what point did you begin to feel uncomfortable?"**
This response uses the tool of clarification. The nurse needs to gather more information about the client's feelings concerning his long history of alcoholism, in order to assess the problem. This response also addresses the client's feelings, using the tool of empathy.

– D. "You need to talk about your long drinking history if you are to recover from your illness."
This is the block of giving advice. Also note that the test-taking strategy of eliminating similar options would be helpful here. Options A, B, and D are similar in that they all focus on the long history of drinking, so none of those options can be the answer.

DRILL #7

7. Soon after being admitted to a rehabilitation unit, a chronic alcoholic client says to the nurse, "I don't really need to be here. My wife and family make me drink. My wife spends all my money. My kid just had an accident with his car that cost me a fortune in repairs." The most appropriate nursing response at this time is:

A. "Tell me more about your wife spending all your money."
B. "How did your son's car accident cost you money?"
C. "It sounds like you have financial difficulties."
D. "Tell me more about your concern about being here."

ANALYSIS #7

Critical Elements

Key words:	See bold print
Client:	A chronic alcoholic
Issue:	The client's tenseness when talking about his long history of drinking
Type of Stem:	True response stem (therapeutic communication)

Eliminate Options

7. **Soon after being admitted** to a rehabilitation unit, a chronic **alcoholic** client says to the nurse, "**I don't really need to be here.** My wife and family make me drink. My wife spends all my money. My kid just had an accident with his car that cost me a fortune in repairs." The **most appropriate** nursing response **at this time** is:

− A. "Tell me more about your wife spending all your money."
This is a block because it focuses on the client's wife and money rather than on the client and his problem. This response addresses an inappropriate issue and an inappropriate person.

− B. "How did your son's car accident cost you money?"
This response also focuses on an inappropriate issue. It addresses the client's child and money problems and not his denial.

− C. "It sounds like you have financial difficulties."
This is a good distractor because it begins with clarification words ("it sounds like"), but it is nontherapeutic because it focuses on money as the issue rather than on the client's denial. Note that options A, B, and C all focus on money or finances. Option D is the different one.

+ **D. "Tell me more about your concern about being here."**
This response is the answer because it uses the tool of empathy, focusing on the client's feelings. Also, note that this response is the only response that addresses the client's denial, which is the issue in the question.

Chapter 6

Learning to Answer Questions that Select Priorities

Recognizing Priority-Setting Questions

The NCLEX-RN Exam Test Plan focuses on the application and analysis of nursing knowledge. Consequently, your nursing course exams as well as the NCLEX use test questions that require decision-making, such as those that involve selecting priorities. These questions are difficult.

Here are some examples of the stems found in questions that select priorities:

- What is the nurse's **initial** response?
- What is the **essential** nursing action?
- What is a **vital** consideration in planning the client's nursing care?
- The nurse would give **immediate** attention to which of the following questions?
- What nursing action receives the **highest** priority?
- Which response demonstrates the **best** nursing judgment?
- Which information is **most** important?

ur Prioritizing Guidelines for Nursing ams

e following table presents quick summaries of four different guidelines you n use in questions that ask you to select priorities.

Guidelines Used to Select Priorities

Maslow's Hierarchy of Needs
Physiological needs come first. When no physiological needs are identified, safety needs receive priority.

Nursing Process
Assessment comes first.

Communication Theory
Focus on feelings first.

Teaching/Learning Theory
Focus on motivation first.

A Practice Session of Questions which Require Priority-Setting

Each of the following questions uses one of the priority-setting guidelines mentioned in the table above. As you read each question, try to determine which of the four guidelines provides the rationale for the correct answer for each question. To do this, you will need to read all of the options as well as the case scenario and stem.

Be sure to use all your new test-taking skills when answering these priority-setting questions. First, identify the four critical elements. Then narrow your choices, keeping in mind the guidelines for selecting priorities. If you are unsure of the answer, try using one of the test-taking strategies.

After you have answered the question, read the Analysis. Note that the **key words** and the **correct answer** are in bold print.

DRILL #1

1. A 64-year-old client is hospitalized with chronic obstructive pulmonary disease. Oxygen per nasal cannula at 2 liters per minute is initiated. When the nurse made an assessment at 3:00 p.m., the client appeared to have made a good adjustment to hospitalization. At 5:00 p.m., the nurse found the oxygen cannula on the floor. The client was angry and said, "It's about time you got here. Where am I? Where is my breakfast?" The nurse should give immediate consideration to which of the following questions?

   A. Has the oxygen cannula been off long enough to cause hypoxia?
   B. Is the client's anger related to being hospitalized again?
   C. Does the client need a clock in the room to keep track of time?
   D. Is the client accustomed to eating dinner very early in the day?

ANALYSIS #1

Critical Elements

Key words:	See bold print
Client:	A client with COPD who suddenly displays confused behavior
Issue:	Immediate consideration of the nursing priority in caring for the client at this time
Type of Stem:	True response stem

Eliminate Options

1. A 64-year-old client is hospitalized with **chronic obstructive pulmonary disease.** Oxygen per nasal cannula at 2 liters per minute is initiated. When the nurse made an assessment at 3:00 p.m., the client appeared to have made a good adjustment to hospitalization. At 5:00 p.m., the nurse found the **oxygen cannula on the floor.** The client was angry and said, "It's about time you got here. **Where am I? Where is my breakfast?"** The nurse should give immediate consideration to which of the following questions?

+ **A. Has the oxygen cannula been off long enough to cause hypoxia?**
This question is a high priority because it focuses on an immediate physiological need. A low flow of oxygen is necessary to maintain the hypoxic drive for a client with COPD. Due to his confused behavior and lack of oxygen for a period of time, the client may be exhibiting signs of acute respiratory insufficiency. Here the priority is a life-threatening situation, and Maslow's Hierarchy of Needs is the priority-setting guideline to be used. Good for you, if you also noticed that the key words "oxygen cannula" appeared only in this option!

B. Is the client's anger related to being hospitalized again?
This is a low priority response because it addresses a psychological consideration as an explanation for the client's behavior. It must first be determined whether or not his behavior may be due to a physiological need. Note that the case scenario also states that the client appeared to have made a good adjustment to hospitalization.

C. Does the client need a clock in the room to keep track of time?
This is another low priority response. This option is similar to option B in that it suggests a psychological rationale for the client's behavior. This reason would be explored only after clarifying that his behavior was not due to a respiratory insufficiency.

D. Is the client accustomed to eating dinner very early in the day?
This is another low priority response. This option is similar to option C because it focuses on the issue of time of day. Using Maslow's Hierarch of Needs as a guideline, physiological needs receive priority. Note that you can also use the test-taking strategy of eliminating similar distractors in this question. Since options B, C, and D all focus on psychological considerations, look for the option that is different.

DRILL #2

2. A client hospitalized with COPD has just recovered from an episode of confused behavior as a result of respiratory insufficiency. At dinner time, the nurse assists the client with the oxygen cannula and raises the head of the bed to high Fowler's position. Then the nurse places his dinner on the over bed table and prepares the dinner according to the client's preference. Which nursing action is most essential before leaving the room?

A. Ask the client if he needs further assistance with his meal.
B. Assist the client with menu selections for the following day.
C. Tell the client that the nurse will return to his room in about 30 minutes.
D. Place the call bell where the client can easily reach it.

ANALYSIS #2

Critical Elements

Key words:	See bold print
Client:	A client with COPD who has experienced hypoxia and confusion
Issue:	The priority nursing action when leaving the client's room
Type of Stem:	True response stem

Eliminate Options

2. A client hospitalized with **COPD** has **just recovered** from an episode of **confused behavior** as a result of **respiratory insufficiency.** At dinner time, the nurse assists the client with the oxygen cannula and raises the head of the bed to high Fowler's position. Then the nurse places his dinner on the over bed table and prepares the dinner according to the client's preference. Which nursing action is **most essential before leaving the room?**

? A. Ask the client if he needs further assistance with his meal.
This option is a possibility because this is an appropriate nursing action; however, it might not be a priority. Remember to review all the other options before making a decision. Which priority-setting guideline is used in this question?

? B. Assist the client with menu selections for the following day.
This nursing action would be appropriate, so it might be a possibility. However, like option A, this option is concerned with the client's meals. Look for a nursing action that would receive higher priority.

– C. Tell the client that the nurse will return to his room in about 30 minutes.
This action is inappropriate. Since the client was confused and hypoxic, his condition would warrant more frequent checks. This action will not provide for the client's safety.

+ **D. Place the call bell where the client can easily reach it.**
This is a high priority nursing action because it addresses the client's need for a safe environment. Because of his confused behavior and restrictions with mobility, providing a safe environment in which the client has access to a call bell is a priority. Here Maslow's Hierarchy of Needs is used as a guideline. If a physiological need is not the issue, then safety needs receive priority.

DRILL #3

3. A client hospitalized with COPD is receiving oxygen by nasal cannula. At 5:00 p.m. his oxygen cannula was found on the floor and the nurse assisted the client with the oxygen cannula and raised the head of the bed to high Fowler's position. At 8:45 p.m., the client tells the nurse that he is feeling short of breath and requests that the nurse assist him in changing position. In addition to repositioning the client, the nurse should give highest priority to which nursing action?

A. Put the client on 15 minute checks.
B. Call the physician to report the shortness of breath.
C. Observe the rate, depth and character of his respirations.
D. Give the client a back rub to help him relax.

ANALYSIS #3

Critical Elements

Key words: See bold print
Client: A client with COPD
Issue: Shortness of breath
Type of Stem: True response stem

Eliminate Options

3. A client hospitalized with **COPD** is receiving oxygen by nasal cannula. At 5:00 p.m. his oxygen cannula was found on the floor and the nurse assisted the client with the oxygen cannula and raised the head of the bed to high Fowler's position. At 8:45 p.m., the client tells the nurse that he is feeling **short of breath** and requests that the nurse assist him in changing position. In addition to repositioning the client, the nurse should give **highest priority** to which nursing action?

? A. Put the client on 15 minute checks.
This is a possibility. Any client with a breathing problem must be monitored closely because this could be a medical emergency. However, this is an implementation action. Checking the client every 15 minutes implies that the nurse has diagnosed that the shortness of breath is not a medical emergency. Which priority-setting guideline will you use in this question?

? B. Call the physician to report the shortness of breath.
This is another possibility, but it, too, is an implementation action. Reporting to the physician implies that the nurse has diagnosed that this is a medical emergency. The question, however, gives us no information about whether this is a medical emergency. What should the nurse do at this time?

\+ C. **Observe the rate, depth and character of his respirations.**
This assessment action receives highest priority in this case scenario. Before you call the doctor, an assessment is needed of the client's respiratory status. This question uses the nursing process as a guideline: before any nursing action is implemented, an assessment is needed. You will see that the nursing process is not just a prioritizing guideline in Chapter Seven but, for now, remember that it can be extremely useful when you are faced with a priority-setting question and always should be considered.

– D. Give the client a back rub to help him relax.
This implementation action may be appropriate, but it addresses a psychological need and would therefore have a low priority. It also does not indicate that the nurse has assessed the client to determine that a back rub would be appropriate.

DRILL #4

4. An elderly client with COPD is admitted to the hospital. While bathing, the client says, "I don't know why I have to be here. Everything around here is a constant reminder of how sick I am." Which nursing response is best initially?

A. "Don't worry. Your doctor will let you go home in a few days."
B. "Why don't you like the hospital? Is it something I said or did?"
C. "If I were you, I'd go to sleep. Tomorrow you will feel better."
D. "Tell me more about what you don't like in the hospital."

ANALYSIS #4

Critical Elements

Key words:	See bold print
Client:	An elderly client with COPD
Issue:	Client's feelings about his illness and hospitalization
Type of Stem:	True response stem

Eliminate Options

4. An elderly client with COPD is admitted to the hospital. While bathing the client states, "I don't know **why I have to be here.** Everything around here is a constant reminder of **how sick I am.**" Which nursing response is **best initially**?

A. "Don't worry. Your doctor will let you go home in a few days."
This response is nontherapeutic because it uses false reassurance and demeans the client's feelings.

B. "Why don't you like the hospital? Is it something I said or did?"
This "why" question blocks communication by putting the client on the defensive. "Why" questions are not therapeutic because they make the client feel like he is being interrogated. The second part of the nurse's response also blocks communication, by focusing on an inappropriate person (the nurse).

− C. "If I were you, I'd go to sleep. Tomorrow you will feel better."
This response is a block because the nurse is giving advice and giving false reassurance.

+ **D. "Tell me more about what you don't like in the hospital."**
This therapeutic response uses communication theory and addresses the client's feelings as well as his concerns. This is the best initial response because communication theory identifies that the nurse should first address the client's feelings. The nurse uses the communication tool of clarification to encourage the client to discuss and explore his concerns about his hospitalization.

DRILL #5

5. In preparing an elderly client with COPD to be discharged, the nurse teaches him to position himself for postural drainage. To achieve success in this teaching program, which information about the client is most important?

A. The type of bed the client will be using at home for the procedure.
B. The amount of time required for the client to change positions.
C. The client's goal concerning his ability to be self-sufficient.
D. The client's ability to move about without assistance from others.

ANALYSIS #5

Critical Elements

Key words:	See bold print
Client:	An elderly client with COPD
Issue:	Critical information about the client needed for planning successful discharge teaching program
Type of Stem:	True response stem

Eliminate Options

5. In preparing a client with COPD to be **discharged,** the nurse teaches him to position himself for postural drainage. To achieve success in this **teaching program,** which information about the client is **most important?**

? A. The type of bed the client will be using at home for the procedure.
This might be a possibility. Maintaining pulmonary function by effective postural drainage is important. A mechanical bed that facilitates postural drainage is very important, however, you should read all the other options to see if there is a more important consideration.

? B. The amount of time required for the client to change positions.
This option is another possibility. Options A and B both concern very specific information, however, so you want to start looking for a more global option that fits the criterion. Continue reading.

+ C. **The client's goal concerning his ability to be self-sufficient.**
According to teaching/learning theory, the client's motivations and goals are a primary concern for success in any teaching program. If a client is not motivated or goal directed, a discharge teaching program is not effective. Note that this option is also very global, in comparison to options A, B and D.

? D. The client's ability to move about without assistance from others.
This option is another good possibility. When selecting between options C and D, however, C is the better choice because the client must first be motivated for the teaching to be effective. The focus of this question is to measure success in a teaching program -- not the effectiveness of postural drainage.

NOTES

Chapter 7

Learning to Answer Questions that Involve Use of the Nursing Process

Your nursing course exams, as well as the NCLEX-RN Exam, incorporate the nursing process as an integral part of the Test Plan, because this is **the method by which one applies nursing knowledge** in the practice of nursing. In Chapter Six, you were introduced to using the nursing process as a prioritizing guideline. In this chapter you will gain additional experience with the prioritizing aspect of the nursing process and you will practice questions designed to test your ability to apply and understand it as well.

Nursing course exams and the NCLEX-RN Exam Test Plan incorporate all five categories or phases of the nursing process: Assessment, Analysis, Planning, Implementation, and Evaluation.

For this reason, when preparing for any nursing exam, it is beneficial to practice answering test questions that involve the nursing process. This is especially true for the NCLEX: on this exam, the questions are equally distributed among the five categories.

In this chapter, test questions are presented that reflect each of the five categories of the nursing process. Follow along in this chapter to review the specific nursing behaviors associated with each category of the nursing process.

ASSESSMENT

Nursing Behaviors Associated with the Assessment Phase of the Nursing Process

- Gathering objective and subjective data
- Identifying signs and symptoms
- Evaluating environments
- Identifying the nurse's reaction
- Verifying data
- Communicating information

When answering questions that focus on the assessment process, keep in mind the following:

- Terms such as "observe," "monitor," "check," "obtain information" or "find out" all refer to the assessment process.
- Remember to **assess first,** before planning or implementing nursing care.
- When assessing, be sure to focus on the **issue** of the question. For example, is it a drug, a disorder, or an early sign of a complication?

A Practice Session Focusing on Learning to Answer Assessment Questions

Read and answer the following assessment questions. Remember to identify the critical elements. When you know the type of stem and the issue, make a decision about each option as you read it by using the selection procedure, keeping in mind the nursing behaviors included in assessment. After you have answered the question, read the analysis. The **key words** and the **correct answer** are in bold print.

The practice sessions on the other four categories of the nursing process require similar problem-solving and test-taking methods. (**Always** identify the critical elements and use your test-taking strategies!)

DRILL #1

1. A client is returning from the recovery room to the surgical unit following abdominal surgery. Upon his arrival in the client care unit, which parameter would be the initial focus of the nurse's assessment?

   A. Urine output.
   B. Vital signs.
   C. Pain in the incision.
   D. Status of the dressing.

ANALYSIS #1

Critical Elements	
Key words:	See bold print
Client:	A client returning after abdominal surgery
Issue:	Initial focus of postoperative nursing assessment
Type of Stem:	True response stem

Eliminate Options

1. A client is returning from the recovery room to the surgical unit **following abdominal surgery**. Upon his arrival in the client care unit, which parameter would be the **initial** focus of the nurse's **assessment?**

? A. Urine output.
This is a possibility, since postoperative assessment of urine output is necessary to measure renal, circulatory, and genitourinary function. However, this would not be the initial focus for postoperative assessment. When answering questions that require prioritizing, remember to read all options before selecting the answer.

+ **B. Vital signs.**
This is the initial focus of your assessment. At this time the nurse needs to gather objective data about the client's condition. This is a critical situation in which it is necessary to implement the ABC guideline. First, the airway and breathing are monitored by observing the rate of respirations. Next, the circulation is assessed by monitoring the pulse rate and the blood pressure.

? C. Pain in the incision.
This is an appropriate assessment and a possible option, but not the focus of your initial assessment. It is necessary to manage and monitor postoperative pain since the greatest postoperative pain occurs during

the first 12 to 36 hours. Potent drugs may depress the respiratory rate and increase tracheal secretions. Management of pain is necessary for client comfort and prevention of postoperative atelectasis and pneumonia, however, this is not the highest priority.

? D. Status of the dressing.
This is another possibility, since it is necessary to observe the dressing for amount, type, odor and consistency of the drainage. Any drainage is marked and noted on the dressing. This is another important assessment, but it is not the initial focus.

DRILL #2

2. The nurse caring for a client who is receiving an intravenous infusion has been monitoring the IV site for signs of infiltration. In assessing an IV site that has become infiltrated, the nurse knows that which finding is unexpected?

A. The infusion rate slows or stops while the tubing is not kinked.
B. The area around the injection site feels warm to the touch.
C. Swelling, hardness, or pain is found around the needle site.
D. Blood fails to return in the tubing when the bottle is lowered.

ANALYSIS #2

Critical Elements

Key words:	See bold print
Client:	Any client receiving IV infusion
Issue:	Signs of infiltration
Type of Stem:	False response stem

Eliminate Options

2. The nurse caring for a client who is receiving an **intravenous infusion** has been monitoring the IV site for signs of infiltration. In **assessing** an IV site that has become **infiltrated**, the nurse knows that which finding is **unexpected**?

– A. The infusion rate slows or stops while the tubing is not kinked.
This finding is indicative of an infiltration. You are looking for a finding that is unexpected in an infiltration. When infiltration occurs, the IV fluid enters the subcutaneous space and the flow of the IV fluid decreases or may even stop. The area around the venipuncture site swells from the tissue fluid. Note that this assessment question has a false response stem!

+ **B. The area around the injection site feels warm to the touch.**
Since this false response stem asks for a finding that is not expected in an infiltration, this is the correct response. IV fluid is cool, which causes the area around the venipuncture site to be cool. A warm skin temperature indicates phlebitis, not an infiltration.

– C. Swelling, hardness, or pain located around the needle site.
This is an expected finding when an infiltration occurs. Swelling occurs as the fluid seeps into the tissue spaces. This is objective data that the nurse would observe when assessing an infiltration of an IV. As the edema continues, the discomfort and pain increase.

– D. Blood fails to return in the tubing when the bottle is lowered.
This is another expected finding with an infiltration. If the IV is patent when the bottle is lowered, the blood in the vein will flow into the IV tubing. When the needle is dislodged from the vein, blood will fail to return in the tubing when the bottle is lowered. This is not the answer, because the question has a false response stem.

3. A client is eight hours postoperative for a transurethral resection of the prostate gland. Which nursing assessment would be an early indication of a postoperative complication?

A. Pain in the operative site.
B. Pulse rate of 88.
C. Output of bloody urine.
D. Oral temperature of 101.8° F.

ANALYSIS #3

Critical Elements

Key words:	See bold print
Client:	A client eight hours post TUR
Issue:	An early indication of a postoperative complication
Type of Stem:	True response stem

Eliminate Options

3. A client is **eight hours postoperative** for a **transurethral resection** of his prostate gland. Which nursing **assessment** would be an **early** indication of a postoperative **complication**?

? A. Pain in the operative site.
This is a <u>possibility</u>; however, pain is expected and normal after an operation. Pain is one of the earliest symptoms that a client experiences when returning to consciousness. The issue of the question, however, is an early indication of a complication. Pain in the operative site does not indicate a complication.

− B. Pulse rate of 88.
This <u>normal</u> finding is not a sign of a complication.

? C. Output of bloody urine.
This is a <u>possibility</u>; however, bloody urine is expected post TUR. As healing progresses, the urine turns to a pink, then light straw color, and is then free of clots. Since this assessment reflects a normal postoperative course, it does not relate to the issue of the question, which is an early indication of a complication.

+ **D. Oral temperature of 101.8° F.**
A temperature of 101.8° F eight hours postoperatively is considered an early indication of a postoperative complication. A temperature that occurs within the first 24 hours after surgery is usually caused by a pulmonary problem, such as atelectasis. Having the client cough and breathe deeply helps expel mucus plugs that cause collapse of the pulmonary alveoli. This option is the only manifestation that is unexpected in a normal postoperative course and is an early indication of a postoperative problem.

ANALYSIS

Nursing Behaviors Associated with the Analysis Phase of the Nursing Process

- Interpreting data
- Validating data
- Organizing related data
- Identifying a nursing diagnosis

Questions that focus on the analysis phase of the nursing process are the most difficult questions. They require an understanding of the principles of pathophysiology, pharmacokinetics, and psychopathology, as well as growth and development. When answering an analysis question, be sure you have correctly identified the issue of the question. For example, the rationale for bed rest for a client with pneumonia is different than that for a client with a myocardial infarction.

Q&A A Practice Session Focusing on Learning to Answer Analysis Questions

DRILL #4

4. A client, age 64, is admitted with a history of myoma of the uterus. She is to have a hysterectomy. In preparing a preoperative teaching plan, the nurse would give top priority to:

   A. Active range of motion exercises.
   B. A rationale for various tubes, IV's, etc.
   C. The need to record vital signs frequently.
   D. Coughing and deep breathing exercises.

ANALYSIS #4

Critical Elements

Key words: See bold print
Client: A 64-year-old client scheduled for a hysterectomy
Issue: Preoperative teaching
Type of Stem: True response stem

Eliminate Options

4. A client, age 64, is admitted with a history of myoma of the uterus. She is to have a **hysterectomy.** In preparing a **preoperative** teaching plan, the nurse would give **top priority** to:

– A. Active range of motion exercises.
This is inappropriate, since passive, not active, range of motion exercises, are usually performed after surgery.

? B. A rationale for various tubes, IV's, etc.
This is a possibility, since knowing the reason for procedures and equipment helps to relieve anxiety. When selecting the highest priority, however, be sure to review all options before making your selection.

− C. The need to record vital signs frequently.
This is inappropriate, since this is a nursing priority, not a teaching priority for the client.

+ **D. Coughing and deep breathing exercises.**
Teaching skills that involve the client's cooperation in the postoperative period are a priority preoperatively. Pulmonary complications are a common postoperative complication. Teaching the client to cough and deep breathe properly helps eliminate mucous plugs that cause atelectasis in the postoperative period.

DRILL #5

5. The nurse is performing a developmental evaluation of a two-year-old boy. Which observation would the nurse consider a good indicator of normal development for this child?

A. Having command of a vocabulary of six words.
B. The ability to walk up and down stairs without help.
C. The ability to dress and undress.
D. The ability to point at what he wants.

ANALYSIS #5

Critical Elements

Key words:	See bold print
Client:	Any two-year-old boy
Issue:	A normal developmental characteristic
Type of Stem:	True response stem

Eliminate Options

5. The nurse is performing a developmental evaluation of a **two-year-old** boy. Which observation would the nurse consider a **good indicator of normal development** for this child?

− A. Having command of a vocabulary of **six words**.
This is not normal. A two-year-old has a vocabulary of about 200 to 300 words. An 18-month-old child has a vocabulary of about 10 words. This is a very difficult question!

+ **B. The ability to walk up and down stairs without help.**
This is a good indicator of normal psychomotor development. An 18-

month-old walks upstairs, but a two-year-old manages to walk up and down the stairs.

− C. The ability to dress and undress.
This is an inappropriate expectation for a two-year-old. This describes an older child of about three to four years old. A two- to three-year-old is only able to undress, not dress himself.

− D. The ability to point at what he wants.
This is not normal communication ability for a two-year old. This describes a one-year-old infant. Because of increased language ability, a normal two-year-old does not need to point.

DRILL #6

6. A client had a cholecystectomy this morning. She returned to the unit eight hours ago. Her temperature is now 102.4° F. Her dressing is dry and intact, she has not yet been out of bed, and she has complained of incisional pain and was medicated with Demerol about 30 minutes ago. What should the nurse do first?

A. Give her Tylenol 650 mg p.o., immediately.
B. Report the elevated temperature to the physician.
C. Do a physical assessment of the client's chest.
D. Send a urine specimen to the lab for culture.

ANALYSIS #6

Critical Elements

Key words:	See bold print
Client:	A client eight hours post cholecystectomy
Issue:	Signs of postoperative complications
Type of Stem:	True response stem

Eliminate Options

6. A client had a **cholecystectomy** this morning. She returned to the unit **eight hours ago**. Her temperature is now **102.4° F.** Her **dressing is dry and intact**, she has **not yet been out of bed,** and she has complained of **incisional pain** and was medicated with **Demerol** (meperidine) about **30 minutes ago**. What should the nurse **do first**?

? A. Give her Tylenol 650 mg p.o., immediately.
This is a possibility, since the client does have an elevated temperature that needs to be medicated -- but is this the priority at this time? What is the issue in this question? What should the nurse do first? Review the other options to see if another action would receive higher priority.

? B. Report the elevated temperature to the physician.
This is a possibility; certainly, this temperature needs to be reported. Again, look at all the answers to see if another action would take priority.

+ **C. Do a physical assessment of the client's chest.**
This action is the nursing priority in this case scenario, because the elevated temperature is a sign of a possible postoperative complication in a client who was immobilized by surgery and a medication. Eight hours after surgery, the nurse assessed the client to have an elevated temperature. A temperature in the first 24 hour period is usually due to a pulmonary problem. At this time, more data needs to be collected about the client's lungs. First, a physical assessment of the chest is needed. After this assessment is made, information about the elevated temperature and the physical chest assessment needs to be reported to the physician. This question requires an analysis of the assessment data and priority setting.

? D. Send a urine specimen to the lab for culture.
This is another possibility; however, a urine infection would occur about 48 hours after surgery and is unlikely at this time. In addition, note that this option represents a medical action and not a nursing action. Avoid actions that are not within the domain of nursing!

DRILL #7

7. An 18-month-old toddler has just undergone a craniotomy. In the immediate postoperative period, the nurse would give top priority to which symptom?

A. Blood pressure of 80/60.
B. Change in the level of consciousness.
C. Depressed fontanelle.
D. Pulse rate of 130.

ANALYSIS #7

Critical Elements

Key words:	See bold print
Client:	A client eight hours post cholecystectomy
Issue:	Signs of postoperative complications
Type of Stem:	True response stem

Eliminate Options

7. An **18-month-old toddler** has just undergone a **craniotomy.** In the **immediate postoperative** period the nurse would give **top priority** to which **symptom?**

A. Blood pressure of 80/60.
This is a <u>normal</u> value for the blood pressure of an 18-month-old. Be sure to know age-appropriate vital signs!

B. Change in the level of consciousness.
This is the initial symptom of increased intracranial pressure and could signal a <u>life-threatening complication</u> after a craniotomy. Behavior changes such as restlessness, fatigue, lethargy, stupor, and coma occur as the pressure increases. This finding necessitates immediate action by the nurse.

C. Depressed fontanelle.
This is <u>not a priority</u>. A depressed fontanelle is evident in fluid loss and dehydration.

D. Pulse rate of 130.
This is a <u>normal</u> pulse rate for a toddler.

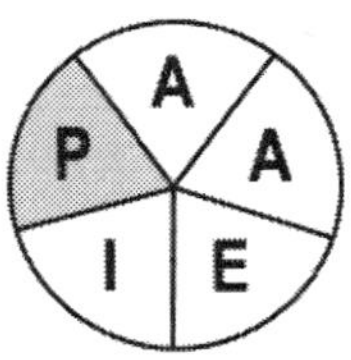

PLANNING

Nursing Behaviors Associated with the Planning Phase of the Nursing Process

- **Developing and modifying nursing care plans**
- **Cooperating with other health personnel for delivery of client care**
- **Recording relevant information**

When answering questions that focus on the planning process, keep in mind the following:

- The answer involves something that is included in the *nursing* care plan, rather than in the *medical* plan. This exam is about nursing, so focus on the nursing action rather than on the medical action.

- When planning specific care, highlight the issue of the question.

Q&A A Practice Session Focusing on Learning to Answer Planning Questions

DRILL #8

8. A client has had an upper gastrointestinal fibroscopy. Which nursing measure must the nurse plan to include in his immediate post procedure care?

    A. Connect the nasogastric tube to gravity drainage.
    B. Keep him flat in bed for two hours.
    C. Have him cough and deep breathe every two hours.
    D. Instruct his wife not to give him ice chips.

ANALYSIS #8

Critical Elements

Key words:	See bold print
Client:	A client post upper GI fibroscopy
Issue:	A necessary postoperative measure to include in the postoperative nursing care plan
Type of Stem:	True response stem

Eliminate Options

8. A client has had an **upper gastrointestinal fibroscopy.** Which nursing measure **must** the nurse plan to include in his **immediate post procedure care**?

− A. Connect the nasogastric tube to gravity drainage.
This is inappropriate. This procedure does not involve a nasogastric tube. In this procedure, a lighted endoscope is inserted to visualize the gastric mucosa.

− B. Keep the client flat in bed for two hours.
This also is inappropriate, since the client is able to freely move around after the procedure. Before the procedure, a sedative or a tranquilizer is given for relaxation. The client is fully awake during the procedure.

− C. Have him cough and deep breathe every two hours.
This is unnecessary and inappropriate, since this procedure does not involve a general anesthetic.

+ **D. Instruct the client's wife not to give him ice chips.**
Of the four options given, this is the only appropriate nursing measure. A topical anesthetic is used to prevent the client from gagging during the procedure, so it is necessary to check that the gag reflex has returned before offering food or fluids. The gag reflex is checked by tickling the back of the throat with a tongue depressor. The gag reflex should return approximately two hours after the procedure.

DRILL #9

9. A child has had a repair of a cleft palate. She is stable and is being transferred to the pediatric unit from the recovery room. Which nursing measure would be inappropriate for the nurse to include in the plan of care for this client?

A. Keep her under close observation for early signs of respiratory obstruction.
B. Position her on her abdomen or side to provide adequate drainage.
C. Use frequent suctioning of the oropharynx to clear secretions.
D. Use arm restraints to prevent her hands or objects from getting into her mouth.

ANALYSIS #9

Critical Elements	
Key words:	See bold print
Client:	A child returning following surgical repair of cleft palate
Issue:	Postoperative nursing plan of care
Type of Stem:	False response stem

Eliminate Options

9. A **child** has had a **repair of a cleft palate.** She is stable and is being transferred to the pediatric unit from the recovery room. Which nursing measure would be **inappropriate** for the nurse to include in the plan of care for this client?

− A. Keep her under close observation for early signs of respiratory obstruction.
This nursing measure is appropriate. After repair of a cleft palate, the

child needs to adjust to breathing with a closed palate. Also, increased mucus secretions may cause obstruction. Remember, this question has a false response stem.

− B. Positioning her on her abdomen or side to provide adequate drainage.
This is another appropriate postoperative nursing measure. Since the suture line is inside the mouth, positioning on the abdomen or side is necessary to promote drainage.

+ **C. Use frequent suctioning of the oropharynx to clear secretions.**
This nursing measure is contraindicated, so this is the answer to this false response stem. Suctioning may injure the suture line. The suture line needs to be protected from injury and infection. Meticulous care is given to drain secretions by positioning, and to irrigate the suture line to prevent infection.

− D. Use of arm restraints to prevent her hands or objects from getting into her mouth.
This nursing measure is appropriate for this client postoperatively. Restraints are used to prevent injury to the suture line.

DRILL #10

10. In preparing to teach a hypertensive female client to care for her health problem, the nurse knows that which goal is inappropriate?

A. The client will exercise moderately each day.
B. The client will maintain weight appropriate for height.
C. The client will discontinue use of birth control pills.
D. The client will eliminate sodium from her diet.

ANALYSIS #10

Critical Elements

Key words:	See bold print
Client:	A female hypertensive client
Issue:	Goal for client teaching
Type of Stem:	False response stem

Eliminate Options

10. In **preparing** to **teach** a **hypertensive** female client to care for her health problem, the nurse knows that which **goal** is **inappropriate**?

− A. The client will exercise moderately each day.
This goal is appropriate. There is evidence that hypertension occurs among people who are in poor physical condition. Remember, the answer must be an inappropriate goal.

− B. The client will maintain weight appropriate for height.
This is another appropriate goal. Excessive body weight causes an increase in arterial pressure. Control of body weight is helpful in reducing hypertension.

− C. The client will discontinue use of birth control pills.
This also is appropriate. Birth control pills and estrogen supplements increase the risk of hypertension.

\+ **D. The client will eliminate sodium from her diet.**
This inappropriate goal is the answer. The complete elimination of sodium from the diet is neither possible nor desirable. It is recommended instead to limit and restrict the amount of sodium in the diet.

IMPLEMENTATION

Nursing Behaviors Associated with the Implementation Phase of the Nursing Process

- Performing or assisting in performing activities of daily living
- Counseling and teaching clients or families
- Using therapeutic communication skills
- Providing care to achieve therapeutic goals
- Providing care to optimize achievement of health goals by the client
- Supervising and checking the work of the staff

When answering questions that focus on the implementation process, keep in mind the following:

- This kind of question asks the nurse to explain, teach, instruct, or respond to the client.
- When identifying a therapeutic response, the empathetic response usually takes priority.
- When giving information about a procedure, keep in mind the accuracy of the information.

Q&A A Practice Session Focusing on Learning to Answer Implementation Questions

DRILL #11

11. The nurse is caring for a very depressed psychiatric client. When approached by the nurse, she says, "Don't bother me. I don't have anything worth saying. Go find someone you can help." Which response by the nurse would be most appropriate?

A. "OK. I'll go now and be back in a half hour."
B. "I have the feeling that I upset you. Don't you want to talk to me?"
C. "I'm assigned to take care of you and I intend to spend time with you."
D. "I would like to stay with you for a while."

ANALYSIS #11

Critical Elements

Key words:	See bold print
Client:	A very depressed psychiatric client
Issue:	Appropriate nursing response to the client's expressions of worthlessness and hopelessness
Type of Stem:	True response stem

Eliminate Options

11. The nurse is caring for a **very depressed** psychiatric client. When approached by the nurse, she says, "Don't bother me. I **don't have anything worth saying.** Go find **someone you can help.**" Which response by the nurse would be **most appropriate**?

– A. "OK. I'll go now and be back in a half hour."
This nontherapeutic response fails to respond at all to the client's feelings and would be unsafe because it results in the nurse leaving a very depressed client alone. Depression is caused by feelings of worthlessness, and leaving the client also reinforces her feelings of worthlessness. Monitoring for suicide is necessary, and leaving her alone would be unsafe. Maslow's theory can be used as a guideline here. Maintaining the client's safety is a priority.

– B. "I have the feeling that I upset you. Don't you want to talk to me?"
This response blocks communication by addressing an inappropriate per-

son (the nurse). The response must be client-centered. Also, the nurse is inappropriately assuming responsibility for the client's feelings. It is not the nurse's fault that the client is feeling this way.

− C. "I'm assigned to take care of you and I intend to spend time with you."
This authoritarian response blocks communication. The nurse-client relationship is built on trust and collaboration. A response that makes the nurse an authority figure is never therapeutic. The focus of the relationship is to encourage the client's decision-making abilities. This response also fails to address the client's feelings.

+ **D. "I would like to stay with you for a while."**
This therapeutic response uses the communication tool of offering self. This response conveys to the client her importance and worthiness. It also results in the nurse's staying with the client, which provides for the client's safety. This very depressed client is at risk for suicide.

DRILL #12

12. A 30-year-old client is admitted to the hospital with chronic renal disease. A two-day-a-week hemodialysis program has just been planned for him. The client says, "Once in a while I have a pain, but I just ignore it and keep on doing what I have to do." In recognizing that the client's statement indicates the use of denial, what should the nurse do next?

A. Respond by saying that he may be avoiding his problem and point out that he does have certain limitations.
B. Reflect his comment by restating his thought in similar but slightly different words and phrases.
C. Analyze his reason for using a defense mechanism and its value to him at the present time.
D. Follow the client's lead and minimize the importance of the physical limitations imposed by his illness.

ANALYSIS #12

Critical Elements

Key words:	See bold print
Client:	A chronic renal disease client
Issue:	Denial
Type of Stem:	True response stem

Eliminate Options

12. A 30-year-old client was admitted to the hospital with **chronic renal disease.** A two-day-a-week hemodialysis program has just been planned for him. The client says, "Once in a while I have a pain **but I just ignore it** and keep on doing what I have to do." In **recognizing** that the client's statement indicates the **use of denial,** what should the nurse **do next?**

− A. Respond by saying that he may be avoiding his problem and point out that he does have certain limitations.
This authoritarian response is nontherapeutic. The nurse is advising the client. Instead, the nurse-client relationship should be collaborative. The nurse needs to help the client resolve his problem by encouraging his self-competency. This authoritative approach destroys the client's capabilities to act in his own interest.

? B. Reflect his comment by restating his thought in similar but slightly different words and phrases.
This might be a possibility; however, a reflecting comment is used to clarify the meaning of the client's statement. The question asserts that the nurse recognizes the client's statement indicates denial, so an additional clarification statement becomes less attractive.

+ C. **Analyze his reason for using a defense mechanism and its value to him at the present time.**
The nurse has already assessed the client's use of denial. What should the nurse do next? The next step in the nursing process is to analyze why the client is using this defense mechanism. This implementation question is a good example of the use of the nursing process in a test question. Note that the test-taking strategy of looking for similar words can also be applied to this question. The idea of "denial" in the stem of the question is repeated in this option by using the words "defense mechanism." This is a very difficult question!

− D. Follow the client's lead and minimize the importance of the physical limitations imposed by his illness.
This inappropriate nursing action would reinforce the client's denial.

DRILL #13

13. An upper GI test is ordered for a client. In preparing the client for this test, the nurse should:

A. Withhold all food, drink, and oral medications after 8:00 p.m. on the evening prior to the test.

B. Explain to the client that the barium preparation she will be asked to drink tastes chalky.
C. Put the client on a high residue diet for two or three days prior to the test to cleanse the bowel.
D. Administer morphine as a premedication about one hour prior to the test.

ANALYSIS #13

Critical Elements

Key words: See bold print
Client: A client who is to recieve an upper GI
Issue: Preparing a client for an upper GI
Type of Stem: True response stem

Eliminate Options

13. An **upper GI** test is ordered for a client. In **preparing** the client for this test, the nurse **should**:

− A. Withhold all food, drink and oral medications after 8:00 p.m. on the evening prior to the test.
This is inappropriate. The client should receive nothing by mouth from midnight the night before the exam.

+ **B. Explain to the client that the barium preparation she will be asked to drink tastes chalky.**
This is the only appropriate nursing action. The barium drink that is used to help visualize the upper GI tract is an odorless, tasteless, but chalky substance.

− C. Put the client on a high residue diet for two or three days prior to the test to cleanse the bowel.
This is inappropriate, since there is no diet restriction prior to this procedure.

− D. Administer morphine as a premedication about one hour prior to the test.
This is inappropriate. A different premedication drug is given for this procedure.

EVALUATION

Nursing Behaviors Associated with the Evaluation Phase of the Nursing Process

- Comparing actual outcomes with expected outcomes of therapy
- Determining impact of nursing actions
- Verifying that tests or measurements were performed correctly
- Evaluating client understanding of information given

When answering questions that focus on the evaluation process, keep in mind the following:

- There may be questions about how the nurse should monitor, or make a judgement concerning, a client's response to therapy or a nursing action.

- Some evaluation questions may have a false response stem. For example, a question may ask for a client's statement that indicates inaccurate information or lack of motivation.

Q&A A Practice Session Focusing on Learning to Answer Evaluation Questions

DRILL #14

14. A client has a long leg cast on the left leg, applied after sustaining a fracture. Which occurrence would suggest that the nurse should call the physician to determine if bivalving the cast is indicated?

    A. The client complains of pressure over the area of the left medial malleolus.
    B. The client complains of severe itching between the left knee and the left ankle.
    C. The client reports pain in the left leg while sitting up in a chair.
    D. The nurse assesses poor capillary filling time with tingling in the toes of the left foot.

ANALYSIS #14

Critical Elements

Key words:	See bold print
Client:	A client who is to recieve an upper GI
Issue:	Preparing a client for an upper GI
Type of Stem:	True response stem

Eliminate Options

14. A client has a **long leg cast** on the **left** leg applied after sustaining a fracture. Which **occurrence** would suggest that the nurse should **call the physician** to determine if **bivalving the cast** is indicated?

? A. The client complains of pressure over the area of the left medial malleolus.
This is a possibility. Complaints of pressure over bony prominences are normal. If the pressure is severe, a window is cut into the cast to alleviate the pressure.

− B. The client complains of severe itching between the left knee and the left ankle.
This is a normal symptom after a cast is applied and does not suggest that the physician needs to be notified.

− C. The client reports pain in the left leg while sitting up in a chair.
Pain is expected after a fracture and when a cast is applied, and during the healing process. Pain that increases in intensity and duration would need to be assessed.

+ **D. The nurse assesses poor capillary filling time with tingling in the toes of the left foot.**
This is a sign of circulatory constriction and requires immediate attention to relieve the constriction. In the evaluation process, the nurse understands that swelling caused by trauma and edema can cause obliteration of blood supply and peripheral nerve damage.

DRILL #15

15. After a myocardial infarction, a client is maintained on a daily dose of digoxin. The nurse is preparing the client for discharge. Which statement by the client would indicate to the nurse that the client needs further instruction?

A. "I should take my pill every morning at breakfast time."
B. "If I feel nauseated, I will take my antacid and go to bed."
C. "If my pulse goes below 60, I should not take my medicine."
D. "I'll start exercising as soon as my doctor says it is OK."

ANALYSIS #15

Critical Elements

Key words:	See bold print
Client:	A client being discharged after a myocardial infarction.
Issue:	Success of pre-discharge teaching
Type of Stem:	False response stem

Eliminate Options

15. After a **myocardial infarction,** a client is maintained on a daily dose of **digoxin**. The nurse is preparing the client for **discharge.** Which statement by the client would indicate to the nurse that the client **needs further instruction**?

– A. "I should take my pill every morning at breakfast time."
This statement by the client indicates an accurate understanding of how to care for his health problem. Digoxin is usually taken once a day in the morning. This statement would not indicate a need for further instruction.

\+ B. **"If I feel nauseated, I will take my antacid and go to bed."**
This statement indicates an inaccurate understanding of potential danger signs associated with his medication and a need for further instruction. Nausea can be a manifestation of digitalis toxicity. Instead of going to bed, the client needs to understand that the nausea requires close monitoring and the attention of his physician. Note the "logic" of this question, which has a false response stem.

– C. "If my pulse goes below 60, I should not take my medicine."
This statement shows that the client understands how to monitor for early signs of a toxic effect of digitalis, and what to do if this occurs. Bradycardia, or a pulse rate below 60, may indicate a toxic effect of the drug, and the medicine should be withheld until the doctor is notified. Digitalis toxicity is a life-threatening situation.

– D. "I'll start exercising as soon as my doctor says it is OK."
Since this question has a false response stem you can eliminate this statement that indicates an accurate understanding by the client. All cardiac clients should consult with their doctor before placing additional strain on the heart by exercising. The amount of exercise is determined by the degree of damage to the heart muscle. This needs to be assessed by the physician.

Chapter 8

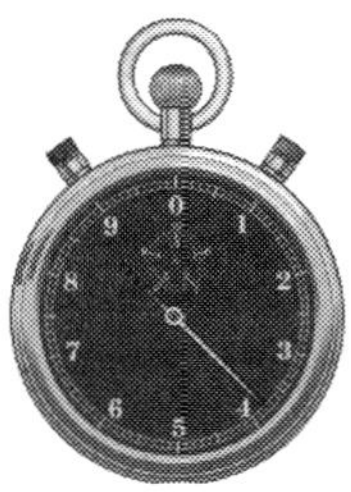

How to Take a Timed Nursing Exam

Pacing Strategy: How Can I Be Sure That I Finish in Time?

If you are often among the last students to finish your nursing exams, then the prospect of taking timed exams can be very stressful. Learning to pace yourself during an exam not only will help you finish the exam in the time allowed, but, more importantly, it will improve your score.

NCLEX-RN candidates should recognize that **good pacing skills are essential for the NCLEX.** This is true, even though most candidates report that they found the allotted time to be adequate and about two thirds of the candidates finish before the time is up. If you are preparing for the NCLEX, practicing your pacing strategy will give you good practice in focusing on test-taking essentials: identifying the critical elements, eliminating incorrect options, and applying test-taking strategies when you are unsure of the answer.

Pacing strategy will keep you from becoming stalled and frustrated when you confront very difficult questions, in addition to keeping you focused on the questions and ensuring that you have enough time to complete an exam. Finally, using pacing strategy to improve your concentration and maintain your energy level will help prevent distraction and fatigue.

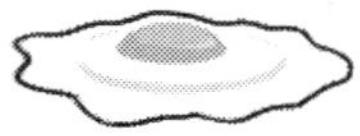

"Once Over, Easy" is a time-saving strategy that you may already know for taking a timed pencil-and-paper exam.

"Once Over, Easy," means that you go through the entire exam the first time, answering only those questions that you can answer easily. After you've answered all the "easy" questions, you return to the more difficult ones.

Unfortunately, it is not possible to skip or return to questions on the computerized NCLEX-RN Exam, but this strategy is still worth practicing and using in your course exams.

The strategy of "Once Over, Easy" is useful because it ensures that you get credit for everything that you are certain you know and about which you can feel confident. In addition, after establishing a pattern of success with the easy questions, you will be better able to correctly answer the difficult questions when you return to them. Often during an exam one question can provide a memory jog that helps you remember information to answer other questions.

When you return to the difficult questions, be sure to use your test-taking strategies. Answer the difficult questions with the confidence that you will be able to correctly answer at least half of them. **Remember that you should not change the answers of questions you previously answered without a very good reason, since your first choice is more likely to be right.**

For NCLEX candidates as well as nursing candidates, the essence of pacing strategy is to plan and monitor how quickly you are answering the questions. This is the best way to ensure that you will be able to answer all the questions in the time allowed.

It is essential to practice using the pacing strategy by answering practice questions in preparation for your exam. Practicing pacing strategy will increase your test-taking speed and accuracy, and will help you fine-tune your ability to use the test-taking techniques and strategies you have learned in *Successful Problem-Solving and Test-Taking*. In fact, using pacing strategy while answering practice questions during your review for the NCLEX-RN Exam is one of the best methods of preparing to take the NCLEX-RN.

Steps for the Pacing Strategy

1. Immediately after you are allowed to begin, check the time. Make sure your watch is working! If not, use the clock in the room. If you are taking the NCLEX, a "clock" will also be displayed on the screen.
2. Determine how many questions there are on the exam, and identify the question that is **ten questions past half way through the exam.** For example, if there are 80 questions, identify question number 50.
3. Depending on how much time you are allowed to take the test, figure out **what time it will be half way through.** For example, if you are allowed 90 minutes to complete your nursing course exam, calculate what time it will be when you are 45 minutes into the test.
4. Begin answering the questions, using your test-taking techniques and your test-taking strategies. On pencil-and-paper exams, skip and do not answer any question:
   a. For which you cannot choose between two choices because they both appear to be right -- and you cannot identify a test-taking strategy to help you decide which is best.
   b. That you do not understand.
5. Write the question number of each question that you skipped on a piece of paper (e.g., at the top of the paper you are given for your math calculations). These questions then will be easy to locate when returning to them.
6. **Try to spend less than one minute per test question. This speed is your goal.** Do not allow any question to immobilize you! Be sure to use your test-taking strategies when you cannot answer a question using your nursing knowledge alone. Make your best selection, and move on to the next question.
7. Check the time. When half the time has elapsed, you should be answering the question that is **10 past half way.**
   a. If you are not yet at that question, you'll know that you must work more quickly during the second half of the exam.
   b. If you are already past that question, you may work a bit more slowly during the second half of the exam.
8. When you have finished going through the exam the first time, go back and answer the questions you skipped. Remember, when you use your test-taking strategies you have a better than 50/50 chance of answering these questions correctly.

NOTE➤ **When studying for an exam, use pacing strategy every time you answer a set of practice questions. Practice is the only way to increase your speed and accuracy.**

What does it take to ace your nursing course exams -- or even to ace the NCLEX-RN Exam on your first try? **Practice, practice, practice!** It is important to emphasize that, as your skill in answering test questions increases, so does your reading speed and comprehension.

Q When I Finish an Exam, Should I Take Another Look?

A Take all the time that you are given! If you find that you finish with time left over, it is suggested that you reread the exam. Perhaps you made an error because you misread something in a question. But remember to change an answer **ONLY** if you have misread the information, or if other questions helped you to clarify information. Otherwise, it is safest to stick to your first answer.

Q What Should I Do If I Keep Changing My Answers When Taking an Exam?

A One of the most unfortunate -- and most common -- problems in taking multiple choice tests is **changing correct answers to incorrect ones.** This causes some students to fail exams.

When answering test questions, always go with your "gut" feeling. This means that you may select an answer for a reason that you are not able to define. You may just like one choice better than another, and it may be difficult to explain why. Trust yourself and choose the answer that you like -- and don't change your answer unless you are sure of your reason for doing so! This principle is also true when taking the computerized NCLEX.

Test-taking anxiety and nervousness are two main reasons why students change answers. When you become nervous while answering a difficult question, this anxiety causes you to lose self- confidence. When you lose self-confidence, even if you have some idea about the question, you feel that you cannot trust your own judgement. Then you end up choosing the opposite of your first hunch or "gut" feeling.

You will increase your self-confidence by answering many practice questions. You can also prove to yourself how many times your "gut" feelings are correct by marking questions answered using this strategy during your practice sessions, and computing how many of these questions were answered correctly.

Q What Should I Do If I Have Trouble Concentrating?

A

Concentration during any exam is crucial. Your ability to concentrate helps you to notice the key words and select the correct answers.

As you learned in the introduction to *Successful Problem-Solving and Test-Taking,* practicing for the test by answering test questions also increases your ability to concentrate. Reviewing in the library, rather than at home, is a good strategy for improving your concentration when answering practice questions -- and you will actually build good concentration habits that way.

If you are nervous and distracted when you are starting an exam, use a relaxation technique and try the first few questions. Students frequently report that after they start answering the first few questions on an exam, they even forget that anyone else is in the room.

As an informed test-taker, you should learn to identify signs of poor concentration. Poor concentration can cause you to misread the test question and answer incorrectly. You need to identify those things that prevent you from answering questions correctly. The following table contains a list of common distractions that you may experience when you are losing your concentration.

Common Signs of Distraction

- You feel a sudden physical discomfort such as a neckache or backache
- You get a real craving for food
- You hear noise from another test-taker (e.g., someone chewing gum)
- You feel extremely tired
- You read the same question many times over
- You listen to someone in the room tap a foot or pencil
- You start to think about your vacation

If you notice these signs of distraction occurring during the exam, take a few minutes to breathe deeply, stretch any achy muscles, and then get back on track. Aim for completing just the next few questions without any distractions. Just as it often happens at the beginning of the exam, concentration can quickly be reestablished and those next few questions can lead seamlessly into the rest of the exam. Refocusing takes just a few seconds. Don't put it off if you find yourself becoming distracted.

Points to Remember

- Pace yourself during the exam.
- After finishing the exam, make use of all the time you have left. Reread the exam.
- Never change answers unless you misread a part of the question, or if other questions helped you to clarify information.
- Be confident! You now have the nursing knowledge and the test-taking skills to succeed.

Chapter 9

How to Prepare for the NCLEX-RN Exam

Your Personalized Review Program

The time has come to review all of the nursing content you have learned up until now. To help you gain control of this oversized task, this chapter leads you through developing your own personalized review program.

Identifying your greatest study needs and focusing on your specific weak areas is an important part of tailoring your personal study program. The basic information we provide may be exactly what is needed by the average student. Some students, however, need more preparation in some areas and less in others. The basic information and tables outlined in this chapter, together with your common sense, can build a personal plan that is best for you. Be thorough in your coverage, and be strict with yourself. The best rule of thumb is not to cut corners.

Students often will cut corners when the amount of material they must review seems overwhelming. It is overwhelming when considered as a whole, "I have to remember everything I learned in the WHOLE course!" Or, worse, for the NCLEX-RN Exam, "I have to remember everything I learned in my ENTIRE NURSING PROGRAM!" The first secret you must learn is one you already know: Divide and conquer. That doesn't mean shave off the corners. It means split it down the middle, and split it again and again, until you have perfect-sized packages for reviewing, relearning, and remembering. The recommendations in this chapter will help you identify how to approach the whole, where to make the cuts, how to package the portions, how to focus on the essential information in each portion and how to budget your time so that you can achieve it all before you take the NCLEX-RN Exam!

We recommend that you study **a minimum of two hours a day, for six to eight weeks before the exam.** For the most part, you will be spending one third of your study time reviewing nursing content and two thirds of your study time answering test questions. Most students feel they need to study as close to the date of the exam as possible, so that they won't forget anything. Your review plan and your study schedule will depend upon your own specific needs and your identification of your own weak areas.

Recommended 8-step guideline for preparing to ace the NCLEX-RN Exam

STEP 1 Identify the "Test Plan" of the NCLEX-RN.

STEP 2 Prepare to Invest the Time It Takes.

STEP 3 Plan Your Comprehensive Review of the Nursing Information Covered on the NCLEX-RN.

STEP 4 Choose Your Review Book and/or Resource Material.

STEP 5 Answer 3,000 Questions Total Before the Exam.

STEP 6 Assess Your Progress.

STEP 7 Review the Steps to Studying Comprehensively.

STEP 8 Document Your Study Program.

You have already made a significant investment in yourself by successfully completing your nursing program. You demonstrated an ability to be committed, dedicated, determined, and motivated. Your next goal is to become licensed! Once you set your mind on this goal, it will be easier for you to follow through with this study program.

Motivation is the key to sticking to your study program and passing the NCLEX-RN Exam. By making the commitment and following your personal study program for the recommended two months, you will successfully prepare for the exam.

STEP 1 Orientation: Identify the Structure of the NCLEX-RN

Remember -- your goal now is simply to **pass the NCLEX-RN Exam.** Therefore, when you plan your review, you should be careful to include **only the essential information needed to pass the NCLEX-RN Exam.**

Although the NCLEX covers all clinical areas, the exam does not test everything that you learned in nursing school! The purpose of the NCLEX-RN Exam is actually rather limited: it is designed to demonstrate whether you are capable of **practicing safely and effectively at the beginning level of professional nursing.** Your review therefore should be focused on what will be on the exam; don't waste your precious review time studying nonessential material.

The NCLEX-RN Test Plan is your official guide to what will be covered. Most beginning nurses practice in the acute care setting. They deal with clients with acute medical-surgical disorders, and this knowledge is what is emphasized on the NCLEX. **The NCLEX-RN Test Plan emphasizes key nursing concepts and is organized according to two major components: the five categories of the nursing process, and the four categories of client needs. These elements of the NCLEX-RN Test Plan are outlined in the following tables. Take a moment now to review these concepts.**

The NCLEX-RN Test Plan
Five Categories of the Nursing Process

❶ Assessment	20%
❷ Analysis	20%
❸ Planning	20%
❹ Implementation	20%
❺ Evaluation	20%
Total Questions	*100%*

Four Categories of Client Needs

1. **Safe, effective care environment 25-31%**
   In order to meet clients' needs for safety, the nurse should have knowledge in such areas as protective measures, personal safety, and control of infection.
2. **Physiological integrity 42-48%**
   In order to meet clients' needs for physiological integrity, the nurse should have knowledge of pathophysiology, drugs, nutrition, emergencies, therapies, and comfort measures.
3. **Psychosocial integrity 9-15%**
   In order to meet clients' needs for psychosocial integrity, the nurse should have knowledge of communication skills, mental health concepts, pathophysiology, treatments, and drugs.
4. **Health promotion and maintenance 12-18%**
   In order to meet clients' needs for health promotion/maintenance, the nurse should have knowledge of growth and development, concepts of wellness, birthing and parenting, and dying and death.

Nursing Concepts on the NCLEX-RN

- **Maintaining the client's physiological integrity**
  About half of the questions will address this concept. It is important to review the medical-surgical area comprehensively.
- **The nursing process**
  The questions will be equally divided among the five categories of the nursing process. It is necessary to practice answering test questions that integrate the nursing process.
- **Nursing threads such as:**
  - **Safety -** Providing a safe environment is an important area.
  - **Communication skills -** This is also a major focus of the exam.
  - Teaching and learning principles.
  - Documentation and accountability.
  - Use of community resources.
  - Clients' rights and confidentiality.

Again, the overall purpose of the NCLEX-RN Exam is to assess your ability to practice safely at the beginning level of nursing, and the primary focus of the exam is the care of clients with acute medical-surgical disorders. These are the areas that need to be stressed when you plan your review.

To plan your review of essential nursing knowledge for the NCLEX, organize the material into the four major clinical areas, which are: medical-surgical, psychiatric, pediatrics and maternity. Then, for a comprehensive review in the medical-surgical and pediatrics clinical settings, use a body-systems approach and group the disorders according to the related body system. **The recommended review sequence is shown in the following table.**

Sequence of Nursing Content for Review

❶ REVIEW MEDICAL-SURGICAL DISORDERS

- Spend the greatest amount of time reviewing medical-surgical content. *Note that 42% of the questions focus on this area.*
- Use the body-systems approach.
- Begin by understanding pathophysiology.
- Identify early manifestations of life-threatening complications.
- Include drugs associated with each disease, and highlight early signs of toxicity.
- Review problems of the aged client with acute medical-surgical conditions.

❷ REVIEW PSYCHIATRIC DISORDERS

- Clarify these disorders, since they cause the greatest amount of confusion.
- Clarify major nursing intervention for behaviors associated with each disorder.
- Identify the drugs associated with each disorder and differentiate between side and toxic effects.
- Identify therapeutic communication techniques. *Note that this is a thread identified in all four categories of clients needs.*
- Review how to communicate with the confused and aging client.

❸ REVIEW PEDIATRIC CONDITIONS

- Use a body-systems approach as it relates to pediatrics.
- Include growth and development, especially of infants, toddlers and preschoolers.
- Identify appropriate play materials at each stage of growth.
- Review acute pediatric conditions in a hospital setting.

❹ REVIEW THESE SPECIAL AREAS:

- Identify current health problems such as drug and alcohol addiction, child abuse, hypertension, myocardial infarction, cancer of the breast, Alzheimer's disease, and AIDS.
- Practice math calculations, especially drip rates.
- Identify therapeutic diets associated with each disorder, and foods included in and excluded from therapeutic diets.
- Review basic safety measures, such as transferring a client from a bed to a wheelchair or cart, administering medications, and walking with a blind client. Note: Safety measures for blind clients is a special thread on the exam.

❺ BRIEFLY REVIEW MATERNITY

- Answer practice questions in this area. Be sure to review the gynecological procedures, such as hysterectomy or radium insertion for cancer of the cervix.

STEP 2 Prepare to Invest the Time It Takes

And it does take time! You will need to set aside the time that is necessary to review the nursing content, and the time it will take to improve your skill in answering test questions.

Perhaps you think that you will not be able to spend much time studying because of all your other obligations and commitments. At this time, it is critical to remember that your goal is to become a licensed professional registered nurse -- and that you can lose potential salary if you fail the NCLEX-RN Exam. You may need to arrange to take time off from work, or hire a babysitter, to achieve your goal. If possible, you also need to put your family or personal problems "on hold" until after the exam. If it all seems overwhelming, remember to start with today. Today, find just two hours to plan your review. Remember, though, planning won't work without your follow-through. **Your priority at this time is to prepare to pass the NCLEX-RN Exam on your first try.**

You can prepare comprehensively and efficiently for the NCLEX if you plan your review carefully. The following table provides a basic two-month time schedule that covers the essential information. Use your common sense to modify the time schedule to meet your individual studying needs. If you feel you have no special considerations, we recommend that you follow the plan exactly as shown.

Suggested Time Schedule

CLINICAL SETTINGS	
Medical-surgical disorders	4 weeks
Psychiatric disorders	2 weeks
Pediatric disorders	1 week
Maternity	3 days
Other areas*	3 days
Total Time:	**8 weeks**

* A minimum of three days' time is planned to cover math and calculations, nutrition, growth and development, and any areas that you find particularly difficult.

After reviewing Step 3, you will have a better idea of any special modifications you may need to make to ensure that your review plan and time schedule better suits your needs. Use the calendar provided in this chapter to plot your personal study plan.

STEP 3 Organize Your Approach -- Plan a Comprehensive Review of the Nursing Information that You Need to Study

As mentioned earlier, when reviewing essential nursing knowledge, it is helpful to organize the material into the four major clinical settings: medical-surgical, psychiatric, pediatrics, and maternity. There are some other special areas to be covered as well. The nursing content that should be reviewed for each disorder for the NCLEX-RN is detailed in the following table. Take a moment to look over these basic review points.

Guidelines for Studying a Disorder

1. **Define the disorder** in the basic terms of the pathophysiological processes that occur.
2. Identify and distinguish between **early** and **late manifestations** of the disorder, and the related nursing interventions.
3. Identify the most important and **life-threatening** complications. (Remember, you are safest when you can assess early characteristics of life-threatening complications.)
4. Determine the **medical treatment** for the disorder.
5. Identify the **teaching-learning** needs associated with prevention of, or adaptation to, the disorder. This includes skills, information, or other help needed to cope.

When you plan your review of nursing information content in the medical-surgical clinical setting, identify the body system where your knowledge is weakest, and begin by studying that body system **first**. Be sure to use the guidelines above to study each body system and its associated disorders.

STEP 4 Choose Your Review Book and/or Resource Material

You need reference materials specifically designed to help you study for the NCLEX-RN. **Class notes are too extensive;** they contain material that helped you to pass your nursing school exams, much of which is not essential for the NCLEX-RN Exam. Your textbooks are also too extensive, and reviewing them all would be overwhelming.

You need to obtain a comprehensive NCLEX-RN review outline book to identify the nursing content and a nursing manual for reference on specific points. Refer to your textbooks only when you need to further clarify information.

In addition, you will also need books of practice test questions (known as "Q&A" books). MEDS, Inc. publishes an excellent NCLEX-RN review book and a Q&A book, as well as a computerized Q&A review. Some suggested materials are listed in the back of this book.

STEP 5 Build Your Test-Taking Stamina -- Answer 3,000 Questions Before the Exam

Answering practice test questions that simulate those found on the NCLEX-RN Exam will help you master the skill of learning to read and interpret multiple choice questions correctly. Frequent practice test-taking sessions offer you the opportunity to perfect your pacing technique and become comfortable using test-taking strategies. Practice questions also enable you to apply your knowledge and give you the opportunity to instantly assess what you have learned. When you answer practice questions, you are:

- Clarifying nursing information.
- Developing your safety judgment.
- Integrating key concepts such as nursing process, communication, documentation, accountability, and growth and development.
- Polishing your analytical thinking skills.

One myth about preparing for the NCLEX-RN Exam is that "the more you memorize, the better prepared you will be." Since the exam focuses on your ability to make safe judgments as a beginning nurse, memorizing facts is only a small part of the preparation process. Most students have the greatest difficulty in **applying** the nursing information to the practice of nursing.

Q&A practice is absolutely essential in preparing for the NCLEX!

STEP 6 Take One Step Back -- Review the Steps to Studying Comprehensively

At this point, you may have a good idea of what your study plan will entail, and you may even have begun following your individual study plan. You could already be well on your way to developing the skills you need to pass!

If you feel that you've come to a standstill, try starting fresh, and make sure you have properly planned your individual study program. Perhaps you accidentally skipped a step, and you got off track. A review of the checklist in the following table should help you get back into alignment!

Checklist to Ensure that Your Study Plan is Comprehensive

	YES	NO
1. Did I begin by using a body-systems approach?	☐	☐
2. Did I pay special attention to the medical-surgical clinical setting?	☐	☐
3. Did I identify the system that is my greatest weakness? Look at the major sections and subsections, and assess your strengths and weaknesses. *Emphasize your problem areas* in your review plan.	☐	☐
4. Did I review the weak areas that I identified in Step 3?	☐	☐
5. Did I draft a brief outline to review content?	☐	☐
6. Does my study plan include answering a minimum of 3,000 test questions (about 100 questions a day)? If you have failed a nursing course; have previously failed the NCLEX-RN Exam; have difficulty with multiple choice exams; or if English is a second language; then you need to answer at least 5,000 questions before the exam.	☐	☐
7. When answering test questions, do I use the strategies presented in this book to narrow mychoices and select the best option when I don't know the content?	☐	☐

STEP 7 Take Your Own Pulse -- Assess Your Progress

Once you have begun your personal study program and start answering practice test questions, be sure to use the following assessment chart to help you plot the direction of your study plan. By using the scale provided below, you will systematically move from areas you have mastered to areas of weakness, until you have covered all areas necessary to build the skills to pass the NCLEX-RN Exam.

Each time you answer questions, calculate and record the percentage of questions that you answered correctly. Also keep track of the number of difficult questions that you initially skipped and then went back to answer, in order to see how many of those questions you answered correctly. **To assess your progress in answering test questions, use the following chart:**

Assessment Scale for Practice Tests

SCORE	RECOMMENDATION
85% +	**Superior!** Don't spend additional time on this area. Feel very confident.
75-84%	**Very Good.** Only return to this area after you have remedied all deficiencies. Feel confident.
65-74%	**Average.** Success in this area is questionable. Repeat until score is above 75%. Keep answering questions, and work on building confidence. You might wish to briefly review the three-step method, just to make sure you are interpreting the questions correctly.
Below 65%	**Warning Signal!** Spend lots of time reviewing this area,and don't cut corners! If you feel that your understanding of the nursing content is adequate, be sure to review your test-taking skills, and then re-test this area using all of the applicable strategies. Remember, test-taking is a skill you can master -- and practice is the best way.

STEP 8 Day by Day -- Document Your Study Program

IMPORTANT! 1/3 of your study time -- review content.
2/3 of your study time -- answer test questions.

In designing your personal comprehensive study program, it is necessary to develop both a daily and a monthly schedule. Review the suggestions in the following table to help you get an idea of what your daily schedule should look like. Studying for two hours a day, eight weeks in a row, must be a planned event! Set up your schedule now -- or it soon may be too late to complete a thorough review.

Your Detailed Daily Personal Study Plan

- **Time and place:** Identify the *exact time* you are going to study. It is a good idea to study in the library, away from distractions, where you will be more productive. Have your study bag packed with all the books you will need. Study when you are well rested.
- **Clinical setting:** Define the clinical focus.
- **Body system:** Begin with the system that is the most difficult.
- **Review book:** Identify the review book that you will use, identify the section to be covered, and keep a nursing manual handy for reference. Only use textbooks when needed to clarify a problem area.
- **Q&A book page number:** Identify the test questions associated with the particular body system.

  Note: Be sure to choose a Q&A book that uses questions similar to those found on the NCLEX and uses the NCLEX Test Plan. You need to practice answering difficult questions that require you to use the nursing process and prioritize nursing actions.
- **Total number of questions:** Try to answer at least 100 questions a day.

Now that you have an idea of the specific nursing content you will cover at on a daily basis, the amount of time required to invest in studying, the resources you will use, and the kinds and numbers of questions you must answer, **use a calendar** to map your plan of attack.

Use the model study program provided in this chapter, along with any personal adjustments, to build a basic personal study plan best suited to meet your own needs. Then, use the calendar provided on the next page to custom design your personal study program.

Fill in the goal you have set for each day of the two months prior to the day you are scheduled take the NCLEX-RN Exam. Use all the information we have provided in this chapter to specify the area to be reviewed and the questions to be answered in your two-hour study period each day in the eight-week calendar. Make sure each body system and every clinical setting is covered.

Be sure to complete your outline and draft your calendar in time to finish your program before you are scheduled to take the NCLEX-RN Exam. This detailed calendar will be your road map each day for the eight weeks prior to taking your exam, providing a daily "To-Do" list to build the skills you need to pass the NCLEX-RN. If you follow the steps we have outlined, you can acquire the skills and confidence that you need to pass on your first try.

Monthly Schedule for Your NCLEX-RN Review

WEEK	MON	TUES	WED	THURS	FRI	SAT	SUN
1	M/S Resp	M/S Resp	M/S Resp	M/S Blood	M/S Blood	M/S CV	M/S CV
2	M/S CV	M/S CV	M/S Digestive	M/S Digestive	M/S Digestive	M/S Digestive	M/S Renal
3	M/S Renal	M/S Renal	M/S Skin	M/S Metabolic	M/S Metabolic	M/S Eye	M/S Ear
4	M/S Neuro	M/S Neuro	M/S Neuro	M/S Neuro	M/S Musculo	M/S Musculo	M/S Musculo
5	PSY	PSY	PSY	PSY	PSY	PSY	PSY
6	PSY	PSY	PSY	PSY	PSY	PSY	PSY
7	PEDS	PEDS	PEDS	PEDS	PEDS	PEDS	PEDS
8	OB	OB	OB	Other	Other	Other	Other

Last but not least, you need to learn about the computerized NCLEX format. Be sure to read the next section of this chapter, and definitely arrange to spend some time in your learning lab using the enclosed diskette if you do not have a PC at home.

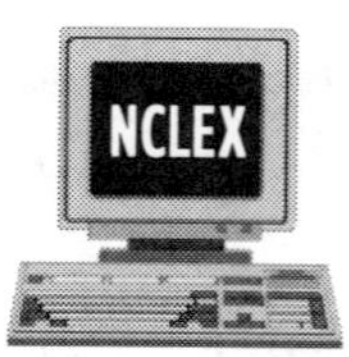

Learning About the Computerized NCLEX-RN Exam

The NCLEX-RN Exam is now computerized. You may see the name of the test written as "NCLEX/CAT-RN" Exam. "CAT" stands for "Computerized Adaptive Testing." The computerized exam "adapts" the exam to the skill level of each individual candidate who takes the test.

How Does "Computerized Adaptive Testing" Work?

The computer contains a "bank" of about 3,000 test questions. When the candidate begins to answer the questions, the computer uses the answers selected to measure the candidate's level of ability -- and then selects the next question at that candidate's level of ability. This process continues throughout the exam.

Adaptive testing is based upon the testing principle that questions that are too difficult or too easy for a given candidate do not measure that candidate's knowledge as accurately as questions more suited to that candidate's ability. The testing continues until a pattern of responses demonstrating a passing (or failing) level of competence is established.

Is This Fair?

Adaptive testing is fair because **the test plan for the computerized NCLEX-RN Exam is the same for all candidates, and all candidates must still demonstrate the same level of nursing competence** in order to pass the exam. As the candidate continues to answer questions, the computer selects questions in all four areas of client needs, using all five phases of the nursing process.

With adaptive testing, candidates with high ability who correctly answer questions at a higher level -- questions that are more difficult -- will not have to answer questions at a lower level. Such candidates can demonstrate their ability to apply their nursing knowledge by answering a smaller number of high level questions. On the other hand, candidates with more average abilities are given the same opportunity to demonstrate their competence by answering a larger number of questions at a less advanced level.

The National Council has done extensive national testing of the computerized NCLEX-RN Exam, and has found that it fairly and accurately measures the ability and nursing knowledge of all candidates.

What Computer Skills Do I Need?

You will not need any special computer skills to take the NCLEX. The exam uses a special color-coded keyboard. To select your answers, you need to use **only two keys** -- and they are **color-coded** to help you identify them easily. The other keys will all be "disconnected" by the program, so that you cannot accidentally use them.

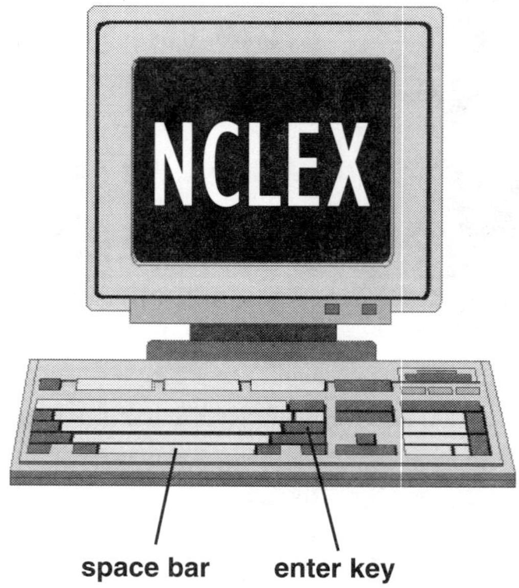

All you have to do is strike one of the two specially color-coded keys to highlight and select your answer, and the other color-coded key to "enter" your selection.

Is There Any Way to Practice Using the NCLEX Computer Format?

Although you do not need computer skills to take the NCLEX-RN Exam, you will be more comfortable and more confident taking the exam if you first practice taking some computerized exams using the same format.

The diskette provided with *Successful Problem Solving and Test-Taking* includes the same questions that are found in Chapter Ten (the "Final Exam"), **but in NCLEX format.** The diskette also includes complete rationales for all correct and incorrect answers, and a special Personalized Performance Analysis feature to assess your progress. If you do not have a computer at home, or your computer will not accept this kind of diskette, you should spend some time in your nursing program's learning lab using one of their computers to practice with this diskette.

What Do the Questions on the NCLEX-RN Exam Look Like?

The exam includes two types of questions: (1) shorter questions presented in a simpler screen format; and (2) somewhat longer questions with more background information presented in a separate **case scenario** (which will appear on the left half of the computer screen) and **question stem** (which will appear at the top of the screen). See the "SCREEN DESIGNS" illustration on the next page.

SCREEN DESIGNS

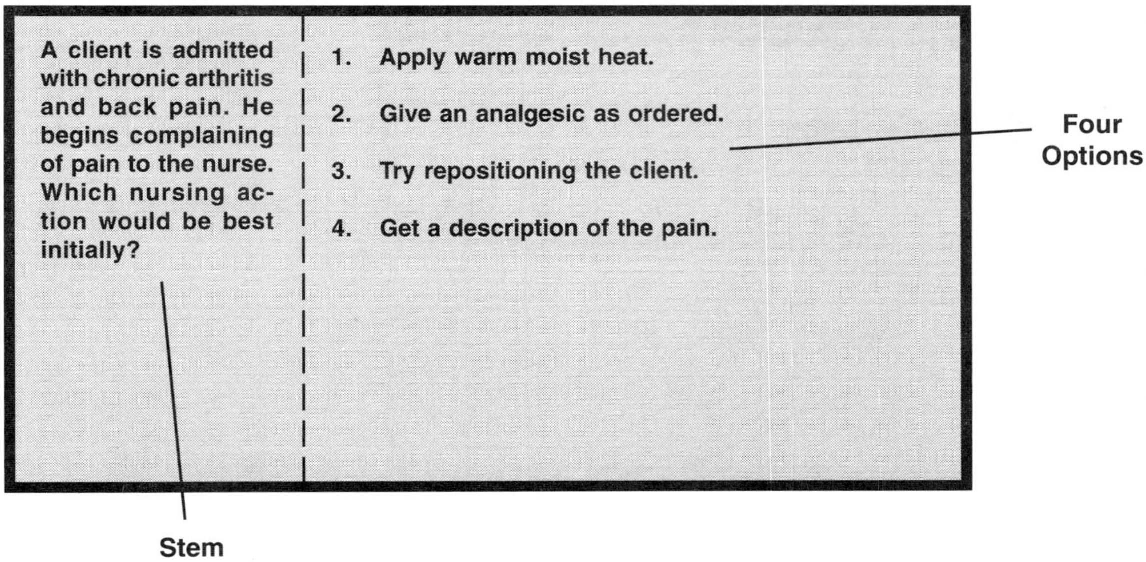

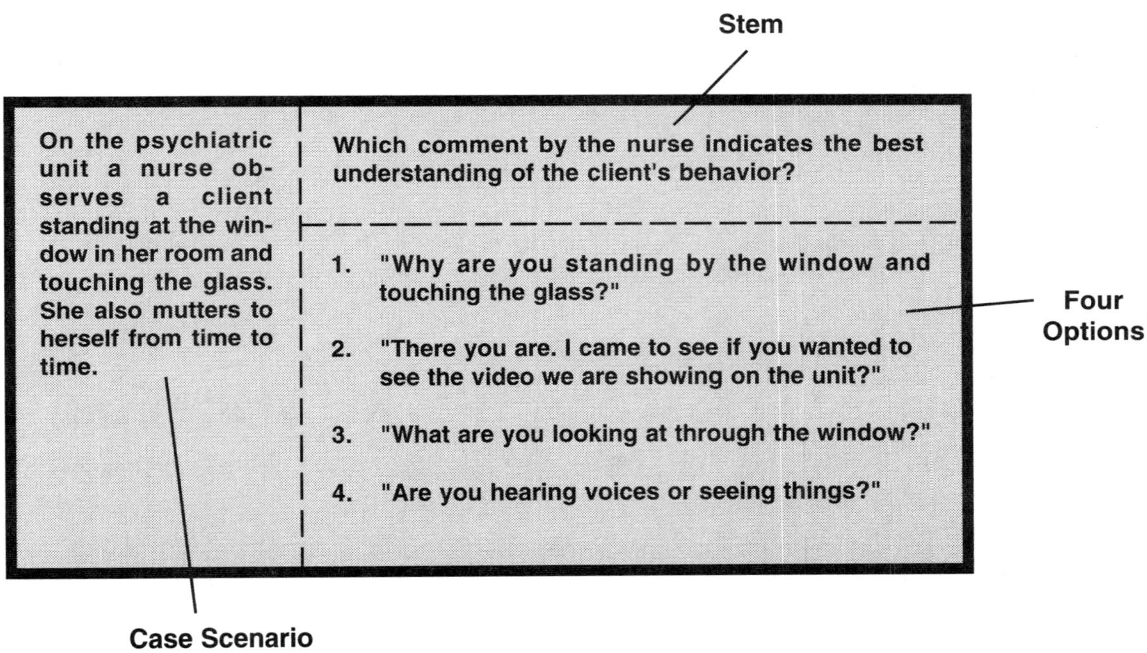

As you can see, the screen separates the **case scenario** and **stem** of the question from the **four options.** When you use the color-coded keys to highlight, select, and enter your answer, the computer records your answer and selects the next question at your ability level. Then the next question appears on the screen.

Q: How is the Exam Scored?

A: The NCLEX-RN Exam is scored according to a weighted formula that takes into account the number of questions answered correctly and the difficulty levels of the questions. There is no penalty for wrong answers, but it is not possible to skip questions on the computerized exam.

Q: How is the Exam Timed?

A: **The maximum amount of time allowed is five hours,** with a ten-minute break after the second hour. Only about one third of the candidates require the entire five hours to complete the exam. A running "clock" appears on the computer screen, so it will be easy for you to keep track of time.

With the new computerized technology, the test can be given year-round and in more convenient locations -- and the test results can be sent to the State Boards of Nursing within 48 hours!

Q: Since the Test Adapts to My Skill Level, Why Do I Need to Use Test-Taking Strategies?

A: You need good test-taking skills to make the most of your nursing knowledge on the NCLEX and achieve a passing score. The test-taking techniques and strategies in *Successful Problem-Solving and Test-Taking* will help you understand the questions better and will keep you focused on what each question is asking.

In addition, because it is not possible to skip questions on the NCLEX, it is very important for you to know some test-taking strategies to use when you are unsure of the answer. When taking a computerized exam, it is important not to become upset if a question is too difficult. Your test-taking strategies will give you some guidelines to follow for difficult questions so that you can improve your chances of selecting the best option and then go on to the next question. Pacing yourself is important, too, to be sure you have enough time to complete the exam.

Comparison of a Typical Nursing Course Exam and the Computerized NCLEX-RN Exam

PAPER AND PENCIL NURSING COURSE EXAM	COMPUTERIZED NCLEX-RN EXAM
Exam setting:	
Administered to entire class at one time, in a classroom or lecture hall.	Administered in small rooms which allow for privacy and quiet during the exam. Sites accommodate between 5 to 25 candidates at once.
Equipment:	
Exam answer sheet, a pen or pencil, and a watch.	The special NCLEX-RN computer, with two special color-coded keys to select and enter answers. No computer skills are needed. However, you should practice answering sample computerized questions before taking the exam, in order to become comfortable with this format. A small "clock" is displayed on the screen.
Scratch paper is provided for calculations.	SAME.
Bring your reading glasses, if needed.	The computer screen is at a greater distance, so reading glasses may not be appropriate for this vision task. Bifocals may also be problematic. If you wear glasses, practice on a computer in your learning lab well in advance of the exam, to determine if you will have difficulty.
Material Covered:	
Covers only specific nursing content covered in one course.	Covers entire range of nursing content, from all clinical areas.
Types of Questions and Test Plan:	
Consists of multiple choice test questions with four options and only one correct answer.	SAME.
Uses the four categories of client needs and the five phases of the nursing process.	SAME.

Comparison of a Typical Nursing Course Exam and the Computerized NCLEX-RN Exam

PAPER AND PENCIL NURSING COURSE EXAM	COMPUTERIZED NCLEX-RN EXAM
May include groups of 3 to 5 test questions pertaining to each case scenario.	Consists only of independent test questions. Most include case scenarios, but each question stands alone and is not linked to other questions.
Number of Questions Asked and Time Allowed:	
All students take the exact same exam.	Each candidate answers questions selected according to his or her own level of ability. No two candidates will take the same exam, but all must demonstrate the same level of competence.
Typically consists of 50 to 100 questions, with a time limit of about one to two hours -- which allows an average of about one minute per question.	Each candidate must answer between 75 and 265 questions, in no more than 5 hours. The computer stops when it determines that the candidate's score reaches (or falls below) the passing standard.
Test-Taking Strategies:	
There is usually no penalty for incorrect answers, so be sure to answer each question.	There is no penalty for incorrect answers -- and you CANNOT skip questions.
Use a test-taking strategy if you can't decide between the two best options, don't know the answer, or don't understand the question. Test-taking strategies are essential to maximize your score. They reduce wasted time and stress when answering difficult questions.	SAME. Test-taking strategies are essential!

Comparison of a Typical Nursing Course Exam and the Computerized NCLEX-RN Exam

PAPER AND PENCIL NURSING COURSE EXAM	COMPUTERIZED NCLEX-RN EXAM
Pacing:	
Do not spend too long on any one question.	SAME.
Save time by leaving difficult questions until the end, and going back to them when you reach the end of the exam if you still have time.	You MUST answer each question, in sequence, and you cannot return to previous questions. However, the questions are selected according to your level of ability.
Requirement for Passing:	
The nursing student must complete the entire exam, and must answer about 66% to 75% of the test questions correctly in order to pass the course.	The NCLEX candidate must demonstrate knowledge above the minimum passing standard by: 1. Correctly answering a minimum of 75 test questions at a high level of difficulty; **or** 2. Answering 75 to 265 test questions with a final weighted competence measure above the passing standard; **or** 3. Achieving a competence measure above the passing standard **for the last 60 questions answered.**
Changing Answers and Reviewing Questions:	
If you wish to change an answer, you may simply erase it.	Answers are "selected" with a special key and can only be de-selected BEFORE you press the ENTER key. Once you enter your answer to a question, you cannot change it.
If you finish before the time is up, you may review the questions when you are finished.	At the end of the exam, you cannot review the test questions.

Comparison of a Typical Nursing Course Exam and the Computerized NCLEX-RN Exam

PAPER AND PENCIL NURSING COURSE EXAM	COMPUTERIZED NCLEX-RN EXAM
How to Prepare for the Exam:	
Review material covered in the course.	The NCLEX encompasses all clinical areas, so you need to plan a comprehensive review.
Use your class notes and textbook for reviewing course covered content.	Use a comprehensive NCLEX-RN review manual, keeping a nursing manual at hand for reference.
Sharpen your test-taking skills, and answer about 200 test questions covering the course material.	Sharpen your test-taking skills, and answer at least 3,000 practice test questions that follow the NCLEX Test Plan.

Test-Taking Tips for the Computerized NCLEX-RN Exam

❶ **Prepare comprehensively** and be sure to be well rested for the exam. This is a vital exam!

❷ **Read each question carefully**, identifying the **critical elements** in the question as explained in this book.

❸ Remember that **each question must be answered, in sequence.** You may not skip questions or go back to change your answer once it has been entered.

❹ **If you have difficulty choosing between the two best options in a test question, be sure to use the three test-taking strategies presented in this book:** (1) Look for a global response option; (2) eliminate similar distractors; and (3) look for similar words in the question and one of the options.

❺ **Use your scratch paper wisely.** Sometimes information from one question may prove helpful in answering a subsequent question. Since it is not possible to return to earlier questions, you may wish to use the scratch paper that is provided for calculations to jot down facts provided in one question that you think you may need in later questions but have trouble recalling.

❻ **Don't panic if someone finishes before you!** The test adapts to each candidate's level of ability. This means that you may take longer to prove that you are capable of practicing competently at the beginning level of nursing.

❼ **Don't panic if the computer stops after a short time!** This does not mean that you failed. The computer stops when the exam is able to determine with at least 95% certainty whether you have demonstrated the ability to practice safely at the minimal level of nursing competence. It is helpful to know that: (1) Approximately one candidate in three will be stopped after about 75 test questions, and more than 50% of those stopped will pass; (2) about 1/3 of the candidates will complete the maximum number of 265 test questions, and about 50% will pass; and (3) approximately 1/3 of the students will fall in the middle of these groups, and about 50% of them will pass.

❽ **Keep a positive attitude!** Remember that you have learned a great deal of nursing knowledge, and that the exam is only designed to determine whether you are able to practice safely and effectively at the entry level.

ATTENTION, ALL NCLEX-RN CANDIDATES!

The best approach to building confidence for the NCLEX and decreasing your anxiety is to get as much experience as possible in taking a computer exam.

If you do not have a home computer, be sure to ask to use the computer in your nursing school's learning lab to take the *Successful Problem-Solving and Test-Taking* "Final Exam." You can also ask your lab instructor to show you some other computerized tests. MEDS, Inc. offers a complete "Q&A" software review which uses the NCLEX screen design and includes useful self-assessment measures. For more information, see the catalog at the back of this book or call MEDS, Inc. at (301) 622-9191.

Chapter 10

A Final Exam

Be confident, and good luck!

Are you ready for the *Successful Problem-Solving and Test-Taking* Final Exam?

You have your choice of using this chapter, or answering the same questions in computerized format using the computer diskette enclosed with this book.

The diskette features the computerized NCLEX-RN screen design, as well as MEDS, Inc.'s unique Personal Performance Analysis to automatically assess your performance. The Personal Performance Analysis classifies your answers to the questions according to clinical area and phase of the nursing process. The analysis also calculates your score according to the critical elements in the question, applicable test-taking strategy, and type of question (prioritizing, nursing process, communication, etc.). If you do not have a home computer that uses this type of diskette, you may wish to use your nursing program's learning lab.

Students who use this chapter in the book for the Final Exam, instead of the diskette, should be sure to schedule some practice time on a computer before taking the NCLEX, to become with the computerized format. To use the exam in this chapter, have a pencil ready to record your answers, and a piece of paper. You will also need a wristwatch, so that you can pace yourself. (The computerized exam displays the time on the screen.)

For a brief review of *Successful Problem-Solving and Test-Taking,* see the "Points to Remember" in each chapter.

To achieve your best score, take this exam when you are well rested. A relaxed, positive attitude helps. Make sure that you haven't skipped a meal. And make sure that you have a comfortable chair.

Tips for the Final Exam:

1. Read each question carefully. If you are taking the exam on paper, circle or underline important words.
2. Be sure to identify all four of the critical elements.
3. Remember that only one answer in each question is correct, and you receive credit only for correct answers. Of the four options offered with each question, you are looking for the **best** one.
4. When you know the type of stem and the issue in the question, make a decision about each option as you read it, by using the selection procedure. Be sure you have correctly identified the client in a communication question.
5. If you cannot decide which option is the best, use a test-taking strategy; if no strategy seems to apply, follow your gut feeling -- and if you don't know, guess! Most exams have no penalty for wrong answers.
6. If you are taking the exam on paper, **be sure to record all your answers!** You may also wish to indicate which questions you answered by means of a strategy.
7. Pace yourself! This exam has 100 questions, so you should allow your self approximately **one hour and 40 minutes** to answer the questions. Find the question that is halfway-plus-ten **(Question 60)**, and try to finish this question at the end of **50 minutes.** Use your test-taking strategies and use your time wisely!
8. If you are preparing for **nursing course exams,** answer the easy questions first, and then go back to the difficult ones.
9. **Attention, NCLEX-RN candidates:** Do not leave any questions blank! Remember, it is not possible to skip questions or return to previous questions on the computerized NCLEX-RN Exam.
10. Concentrate during the exam, and be sure to use relaxation techniques as needed.

Good luck! Turn the page (or log on to your computer and see the instructions on the diskette), and begin.

1. **The nurse visits a client at home one week following his discharge after a myocardial infarction. He is taking chlorothiazide (Diuril) 500 mg daily and digoxin (Lanoxin) 0.25 mg daily. The nurse should give top priority to assessing the client's knowledge related to:**

    1. Sources of potassium.
    2. Sources of sodium.
    3. Activity restrictions.
    4. Signs of a heart attack.

2. **A adolescent client is to have a water system heating device ("K-Pad"), applied to a pulled muscle. The client tells the nurse that the device does not feel very warm. The most appropriate nursing action is to:**

    1. Tell the client that these heating devices never feel hot.
    2. Check the temperature setting on the heating unit and feel the pad for warmth.
    3. Call the appropriate repair department and have them fix the unit.
    4. Turn the temperature up on the unit if it doesn't feel warm enough to the client.

3. **A 34-year-old client who weighs 288 pounds says to the nurse, "I'm going to have surgery and have my stomach stapled in order to lose weight. I've tried everything else, and nothing seems to work." Which response by the nurse would be therapeutic?**

    1. "That's a pretty drastic measure. Are you sure that is what you want to do?"
    2. "I hear that the surgery is only a temporary measure, and if you have the staples removed you will only gain the weight back again."
    3. "It must be difficult to be overweight and not able to lose weight. What does your husband think about the surgery?"
    4. "Can you tell me about the possible consequences and side effects of this type of surgery?"

4. **The nurse finds an elderly client standing in a puddle of water in the hallway of the unit. The nurse does not know this client. What should the nurse do first?**

    1. Ask the client for her name and room number.
    2. Wipe up the water until the floor is completely dry.
    3. Call the supervisor for assistance in identifying the client.
    4. Have the client wait in the lounge until security arrives.

5. **The nurse caring for a client on the evening before his scheduled left below-the-knee amputation provides preoperative teaching, including deep breathing and coughing. Which question would be most helpful for the nurse to ask the client, to evaluate the effectiveness of the preoperative teaching?**

    1. "Do you understand what we have just discussed about deep breathing and coughing?"
    2. "Do you think that you will need to have a sedative to help you sleep tonight?"
    3. "Will you demonstrate for me the correct method of deep breathing and coughing?"
    4. "Do you have any questions concerning your scheduled surgical procedure?"

6. **The nurse is conducting a preoperative interview three days prior to admitting a seven-year-old female for tonsillectomy. The child's mother requests information to prepare her daughter for hospitalization. The nurse knows that the child was hospitalized last year for a fractured femur. Which nursing actions would best meet this child's needs for preparation?**

    1. Suggest a role play, and provide materials.
    2. Remind the child of the experience of her past hospitalization.
    3. Read the child a story about another child having a similar operation.
    4. Tell the child she is only going in to have her throat checked.

7. **A client is admitted to the hospital in respiratory distress. The doctor orders oxygen via mask and the client to be placed in Fowler's position. Which nursing action is most important for this client at this time?**

    1. Support and align the hands with the forearms.
    2. Use handrolls.
    3. Raise the head of the bed to allow for greater lung expansion.
    4. Support the feet at right angles to the lower legs.

8. **A 23-year-old gravida 1, para 0 is admitted to the hospital at 38 weeks gestation with pregnancy induced hypertension. Which finding would the nurse identify as inconsistent with the admitting diagnosis?**

    1. 3+ protein in the urine.
    2. Deep tendon reflexes of +1.
    3. Blood pressure of 148/98.
    4. 1+ pitting sacral edema.

9. **When the nurse enters a client's room, the client's son tells the nurse, "You people can't do anything right. Ever since my father was admitted to this hospital, it has been one mistake after another. I am taking him out of here before you kill him." The nurse's most helpful response to the son is:**

    1. "You feel that your father is not being well cared for?"

2. "We have the best intentions for the clients."
3. "I'll get the supervisor for you."
4. "Your father hasn't complained about the care. What specifically is the problem?"

10. After a myocardial infarction, which vital signs assessment should the nurse recognize as possible indications of cardiogenic shock?

1. BP - 180/100, P - 90, irregular.
2. BP - 130/80, P - 100 regular.
3. BP - 90/50, P - 50 regular.
4. BP - 80/60, P - 110, irregular.

11. An 18-year-old client is hospitalized for treatment of severe depression. Which nursing approach should be included in the plan of care for this client?

1. Giving the client choices.
2. Spending time with the client.
3. Providing a chess game.
4. Encouraging decision-making.

12. A two-year-old is hospitalized with bacterial pneumonia. The nurse will monitor her respiratory status closely. Which signs/symptoms would the nurse identify as the earliest indication of respiratory difficulty?

1. Respiratory rate of 40 to 48.
2. Blood pressure of 80/60.
3. Cyanosis of mucous membranes.
4. Circumoral/periorbital pallor.

13. A client is in labor and is admitted with a blood pressure of 86/52. She is four centimeters dilated and uncomfortable. The nurse should give immediate consideration to which nursing action?

1. Call the physician to report the blood pressure.
2. Turn the client on her side and retake her blood pressure.
3. Reassure the client that everything is all right.
4. Ask the client if she would like some pain medication.

14. During a client's postoperative recovery from an ileostomy, the nurse begins teaching her stoma care. The client refuses to look at her ostomy and tells the nurse, "I'd rather be dead than have to live with this all my life." The appropriate nursing response is:

1. "I can't imagine what you must be feeling; it must be awful."
2. "I'll call your physician and see if something can be ordered to help you to relax."
3. "There's no reason to feel like that. Things will get better."
4. "You appear upset. Would you like to talk?"

15. A client was hospitalized for major depression and treated with nortriptyline (Pamelor). As the client is preparing for discharge, which statement by the client would indicate to the nurse that she needs further instruction?

1. "I'm glad this medicine helps me. My husband and I would like to start our family as soon as possible."
2. "If I should feel hopeless and suicidal again, I have the telephone number of my therapist to call for help."
3. "I hope I will not have to continue taking medicine forever. I guess I'll have to see how I do."
4. "I plan to see my psychiatrist regularly. She told me if I continue to do well, I can probably stop taking my medication in nine to 12 months."

16. A 22-year-old client has had surgery on his foot and has just been returned to his room from the recovery room. The initial assessment indicates that he is stable. An hour later, his roommate turns on the call light and tells the nurse that the client has gotten up and hopped on one foot to the bathroom, using his IV pole for support. Which action should the nurse take initially to provide for the client's safety?

1. Open the bathroom door to assess if the client is okay.
2. Assist the client in ambulating back to bed and get him a urinal.
3. Explain to the client that it is not safe for him to be hopping around on one foot.
4. Get a wheelchair and help the client back to bed when he is done in the bathroom.

17. A 77-year-old client was hospitalized for observation after a fall that he experienced when he was walking for exercise. He is to ambulate for the first time since his fall. He tells the nurse that he is afraid to get up. The best response by the nurse is:

1. "There is nothing to be afraid of. The order wouldn't have been written if your doctor didn't think that you were ready."
2. "Tell me what concerns you about getting up today."
3. "I will have another person here to help you when you get up."
4. "Are you afraid of falling again?"

18. To safely assess for correct placement of a nasogastric tube, the nurse should:

1. Instill 30 ml of saline to assess client tolerance.
2. Instill 10 ml of air into the tube and listen for gurgling sounds with a stethoscope over the gastric area.
3. Aspirate stomach contents with a syringe.
4. Place the end of the tube in water to assess for bubbling.

19. A psychiatric client is re-hospitalized after discontinuing her medication of her own accord. She has responded well to the support of the nurse-client relationship. The client's discharge plans include living with her parents and attending a job training program during the day. What is the most important goal for her remaining sessions with the nurse?

1. Reinforce the importance of taking her medications as prescribed.
2. Anticipate future problems and how she might handle them.
3. Terminate the nurse-client relationship.
4. Promote the client's self-confidence.

20. The nurse knows that the discharge teaching is successful for a client with Hepatitis A virus if the client indicates that she will never:

1. Donate blood.
2. Eat fried foods.
3. Vacation in a foreign country.
4. Order a salad in a restaurant.

21. A 55-year-old client is hospitalized following myocardial infarction. When transferring the client from a cart to his bed, the priority nursing action is to:

1. Have the client place his arms on his chest.
2. Lock the wheels on the cart and the bed.
3. Have at least four people to help with the transfer.
4. Use a draw sheet to move the client.

22. The nurse understands that which statement about reality testing is inaccurate?

1. It is an ego function.
2. It is impaired in psychotic individuals.
3. It is impaired in persons who are mentally retarded.
4. It is the capacity to distinguish thoughts, feelings, fantasies, and other experiences that originate inside the individual from those that are part of the outside environment.

23. The client is to receive a medication for control of tachycardia and an irregular heart rate. The nurse obtains the following vital signs prior to administering this medication: blood pressure 98/54, pulse 48, respirations 30, and temperature 98° F. The client's skin is cool, with cyanosis of the fingers and lips. The appropriate nursing action is to:

1. Administer the medication as ordered by the physician.
2. Omit the medication for a day or two, depending on the client's response and symptoms.
3. Notify the physician concerning the client's status before administering the medication.
4. Give the client one half of the ordered dose.

24. The nurse is preparing a teaching plan for a client being discharged following major abdominal surgery. The client will be doing her own dressing changes at home. Which technique is the most important for the nurse to include in the discharge teaching plan?

1. Opening bandages properly to maintain their sterility.
2. Maintaining strict aseptic technique.
3. Proper gloving technique.
4. Good handwashing technique.

25. A premature infant weighed only three pounds and seven ounces at birth. Following a lengthy stay in the hospital, her weight has increased to five pounds. She will be discharged soon. Which statement by the mother would indicate to the nurse that additional teaching is needed?

1. "My baby is so fragile that I will need to be very careful about everything that I do for her."
2. "I know that my baby will need to see the doctor regularly for awhile, and I have the appointments on my calendar."
3. "My mother is going to stay with me for several weeks to help me with my older children."
4. "I have the nursery, clothing, bottles, and diapers all ready for the day we bring our baby home."

26. A client was told by her doctor that a lump was found in her breast and that a biopsy would have to be done. The client asks the nurse, "Do you think it is cancer?" Which nursing response is best initially?

1. "You seem to be worried about what the doctor may find."
2. "Do you have a family history of breast cancer?"
3. "We won't know anything until the biopsy is done."
4. "Most lumps are not cancerous, so you really shouldn't worry."

27. A client has been told by the doctor that he has cancer and that it has advanced so far that treatment will not help. When the nurse enters the room to set up his bath equipment, he says to the nurse, "I'm not an invalid, you know. I can take care of myself. Get out and leave me alone." What is the best nursing response?

1. "I know that you are not an invalid. I was just trying to help you."
2. "It sounds to me like you are angry about something. Did somebody do something wrong?"
3. "You are pretty upset. Let's talk about it."
4. "I'll just set up this equipment for you to bathe and come back later when you're not so angry."

28. A six-year-old male is admitted with a spiral fracture of the humerus and multiple bruises of the forearm. The physician states that the injuries and other signs are suspicious for abuse. The nurse's initial goal is to:

1. Prevent further abuse of the client.
2. Encourage the client to express his feelings.
3. Determine who is responsible for the abuse.
4. Teach the parents the appropriate methods of discipline.

29. While caring for a client, the nurse should practice good body mechanics and avoid muscle strain. In using good body mechanics, the nurse would avoid:

1. Moving muscles quickly, using short tugs.
2. Using the longest and strongest muscles of the body.
3. Leaning toward objects being pushed, such as a stretcher.
4. Carrying objects close to the body without touching your clothing.

30. An elderly client is admitted to the hospital with pneumonia. His daughter, who takes care of him at home, says to the nurse, "I'm so glad he is here. You can take much better care of him than I can." The best nursing response to the daughter is:

1. "We do have the equipment and people to take care of sick clients."
2. "It is not easy to care for the elderly. How do you manage?"
3. "Sir, your daughter takes good care of you at home, doesn't she?"
4. "Are you feeling guilty because your father has pneumonia?"

31. A client has pregnancy induced hypertension. In planning care for this client prior to delivery, which is most the most essential nursing order?

1. Assess fluid balance hourly and maintain optimum placental perfusion.
2. Monitor urine output and assure a brief rest period every shift.
3. Check the blood pressure before and after each time the client is out of bed.
4. Observe for amount of edema and provide for diversionary activities.

32. A 22-year-old client sustained a T-4 spinal cord injury. While doing morning assessments four weeks post-injury, the nurse discovers his BP is 280/140 and he is complaining of nasal stuffiness and a severe, pounding headache. The first nursing action is to:

1. Sit the client upright.
2. Call the physician.
3. Check the client's bladder for distension.
4. Administer the prescribed antihypertensive.

33. A client is in the hospital with renal failure. She is on fluid restriction. Which nursing measure is inappropriate?

1. Provide a variety of fluids in small containers.
2. Inform the client and family about the restriction.
3. Allow the client to help keep a record of oral intake.
4. Provide fluids only during meal times.

34. The physician has ordered the client to be discharged on a 2000 calorie diabetic diet. What is the most important nursing action in developing a teaching plan for this client's diet?

1. Obtain sample menus from the dietician to give to the client.
2. Ask the client to identify the types of foods that she usually eats and prefers.
3. Tell the client that she will have to change all of her previous eating habits.
4. Advise the client to buy only dietetic foods.

35. An eight-year-old client was admitted to the hospital with a diagnosis of acute rheumatic fever. Immediately after admission, which nursing assessment is most important?

1. Auscultation of the rate and characteristics of heart sounds.
2. Determining the location and severity of joint pain.
3. Identifying the degree of anxiety related to the diagnosis.
4. Determining the family's emotional and financial needs.

36. A client recently diagnosed with multiple sclerosis questions the nurse concerning the usual course of the disease. What would be the most appropriate response by the nurse?

1. "Each client is different. We cannot tell what will happen."
2. "I can see that you are worried, but it's too soon to predict what will happen."
3. "Usually, acute episodes are followed by remissions, which may last a long time."
4. "It's too early to think about the future; let's focus on the present and go day-by-day."

37. While transferring a client with left-leg weakness from the bed to a wheelchair, the priority nursing action is to:

1. Have the seat of the wheelchair at a right angle to the bed.

2. Lock the wheels on the bed and the wheelchair.
3. Allow the client to do as much as possible to increase his sense of independence.
4. Have the client lock his hands around the nurse's neck to provide the client with a sense of security.

38. The nurse enters the room and finds a mother crying. Her son has been diagnosed with leukemia and is currently receiving chemotherapy. The mother says, "I just can't believe he's going to lose all his beautiful blonde hair!" Which response by the nurse is most justifiable?

1. "Sometimes the hair only thins."
2. "You're feeling a lot of loss right now."
3. "Remember, hair loss means the chemotherapy is working!"
4. "Kids love to wear the special baseball caps we have."

39. A client says to the nurse, "I am so frustrated with having five kids. My husband won't do anything to help me keep from getting pregnant." Which is the best nursing action initially?

1. Refer the client and spouse to family planning services.
2. Find out if the client could use a contraceptive that would not involve her husband.
3. Assess what the client means by "being frustrated."
4. Ask the client if her husband is interested in birth control.

40. An adult client is diagnosed with pneumonia and is being treated with penicillin G sodium 3 million units IV every four hours. When completing the drug history, it is especially important for the nurse to assess the client for allergies to which medications?

1. Antituberculars.
2. Calcium channel blockers.
3. Aminoglycosides.
4. Cephalosporins.

41. A client is gravida 5 para 4. During admission, the nurse assesses that contractions are occurring every two minutes and lasting approximately 45 seconds. The client says she has been in labor for approximately 10 hours. The priority assessment the nurse needs to make at this time is:

1. Time the client last ate.
2. Cervical dilatation.
3. Allergies to medications.
4. Vital signs.

42. A client is admitted to the hospital at 38 weeks of gestation with a large amount of bright red vaginal bleeding. A diagnosis of partial abruptio placenta is made. She is on the fetal monitor, and her vital signs are: FH 138 regular, BP 98/52, pulse 118, respirations 24, temperature 97.6° F. Assuming all of the following are ordered by the physician, the nurse should give first priority to which nursing action?

1. Abdominal-perineal prep.
2. Insert Foley catheter.
3. Sign informed consent for surgery.
4. Start an IV.

43. A 15-year-old client is being seen in the family planning clinic. She says to the nurse that she is nervous and has never had a pelvic examination before. The appropriate response by the nurse is:

1. "All you have to do is relax."
2. "It is only slightly uncomfortable."
3. "What part of the exam makes you nervous?"
4. "If you want birth control pills, then a pelvic exam is required."

44. The first, most important nursing action when a nurse discovers a fire in a client's room is to:

1. Pull the fire alarm and notify the hospital operator.
2. Close fire doors and client room doors.
3. Remove the client from the room.
4. Place moist towels or blankets at the threshold of the door of the room with the fire.

45. In assessing an adult client with diabetes mellitus, the nurse would identify which finding as unexpected with this diagnosis?

1. Possible increased body weight.
2. Increased urinary output.
3. Periods of polydypsia.
4. Altered heart rate and rhythm.

46. A client is to be up in a chair three times a day. He is paralyzed from the waist down. What is the best nursing approach when transferring the client from a bed into a wheelchair?

1. Place the wheelchair close to the foot of the bed.
2. Utilize the principles of body mechanics while providing a safe transfer for the client.
3. Slide the client to the edge of the bed, keeping the nurse's back straight and using a rocking motion to pull the client.
4. Place the nurse's arms under the client's axillae from the back of the client.

47. A client puts her call light on and tells the nurse that she has to urinate. The client has had a Foley catheter in place since her surgery two days ago. Which is the most appropriate nursing action initially?

1. Remind the client that she has a Foley catheter in place and does not need to go to the bathroom.
2. Replace the Foley catheter with a new catheter.
3. Explain to the client that the urge to void is a common occurrence for clients who have urinary catheters.
4. Check the catheter and tubing for kinks and note the urine output in the drainage bag.

48. A 49-year-old client has been diagnosed with iron deficiency anemia. When teaching the client about her diet, the nurse should recommend an increased intake of:

1. Fresh fruits.
2. Milk and cheese.
3. Organ meats.
4. Whole grain breads.

49. A client is to have a nasogastric tube inserted because of an obstruction in his bowel. The nurse explains the procedure to him and is about to begin the insertion, when the client says, "No way! You are not putting that hose down my throat. Get away from me." The best nursing response is:

1. "You have the right to refuse treatment. Why don't you talk to your doctor about it?"
2. "Something is upsetting you. Can you tell me what it is?"
3. "What exactly do you feel about this 'hose'?"
4. "It'll be easier for you to just get it over with. It only gets harder if you get worked up over it and you won't get better without this tube."

50. The nurse tells a client that the doctor has ordered an intravenous line to be started. The client appears to be upset but says nothing to the nurse. Which is the best nursing response?

1. "Do you have any questions about the procedure?"
2. "The doctor wants you to have antibiotics, and this method eliminates getting frequent injections."
3. "What is there about this procedure that concerns you?"
4. "It only hurts a little bit. It'll be over before you know it."

51. A client shows the nurse the result of his recent tuberculin skin test. The site is red and swollen. The nurse interprets this as:

1. The client has active tuberculosis.
2. The client has a history of tuberculosis.
3. The tubercle bacillus is in the active pulmonary stage of tuberculosis.
4. The client has had contact with the tubercle bacillus.

52. A client is in the hospital and has weakness on her left side because of a stroke. She becomes upset when eating because liquids drool out of her mouth on her weak side. What nursing intervention would be most appropriate?

1. Provide only pureed and solid foods to prevent drooling, in order to prevent the client from becoming upset.
2. Have a member of the family assist with the client's feedings.
3. Teach the client how to drink fluids on the unaffected side to prevent drooling.
4. Have the client use a syringe to squirt liquids into the back of her mouth.

53. A 10-year-old boy is in sickle cell crisis. Which nursing action is contraindicated?

1. Administer oxygen via nasal cannula as prescribed.
2. Encourage the client to increase oral fluid intake.
3. Administer narcotics only for very severe pain.
4. Encourage as much exercise as possible during the crisis.

54. A 21-year-old client has sustained a basal skull fracture. The nurse notices drainage from his right nostril. The priority nursing action is to:

1. Notify his physician.
2. Suction his nostril.
3. Test the drainage for glucose.
4. Ask the client to blow his nose.

55. If verapamil hydrochloride (Calan) is administered with propranolol (Inderal), the nurse should monitor the client closely for signs of:

1. Hypertension.
2. Increased peripheral resistance.
3. Bradycardia and heart failure.
4. Diarrhea.

56. In assessing a client after a bronchoscopy, the nurse would give immediate attention to:

1. Blood-tinged mucous.
2. Complaints of hoarseness when speaking.
3. Irritation and discomfort when swallowing.
4. Difficulty breathing.

57. The nurse is caring for a client who had abdominal surgery two days ago. Which assessment data requires immediate action by the nurse?

1. A urinary drainage bag with 100 ccs in a two-hour period.
2. A wound dressing with thick light green drainage.
3. A blood pressure reading of 98/66.
4. Shallow respirations, with a rate of 26.

58. A depressed client and her husband attend a client education class on the topic of depression and learn about the behaviors that could indicate a recurrence of depression. To evaluate the effectiveness of the teaching, the nurse asks the client to identify the indications of recurrence of depression. Which behavior or symptom if named by the client would indicate to the nurse that the client requires further instruction?

1. Psychomotor retardation.
2. Grandiosity.
3. Self-devaluation.
4. Insomnia.

59. An 18-month-old girl is admitted for a surgical repair of the cleft palate. She returns from the operating room supine, with an IV and a mist tent on room air. Which is the priority nursing action?

1. Medicate for pain.
2. Check the IV for signs of infiltration.
3. Turn the child on her side.
4. Review the postoperative orders.

60. A male nurse received a doctor's order to catheterize one of his female clients. The client says, "I'm not going to allow a male nurse to catheterize me." The appropriate response by the nurse is:

1. "Your doctor is a male. Would you let him catheterize you?"
2. "I've done this many times with no problems."
3. "You can explain to your doctor why the catheter wasn't inserted."
4. "You appear to be upset. Let me find a female nurse to help with the procedure."

61. A confused elderly client is found wandering around the ward wearing a bathrobe and cotton socks. He is bumping into walls as he walks. At this time, the nurse should:

1. Take the client's shoes to him and assist him in putting them on.
2. Accompany the client to his room and obtain a baseline assessment.
3. Ask the client to return to his room and rest until he feels better.
4. Tell the client to be careful of any wet spots on the floor.

62. A client, age 31, is brought to the Emergency Room after an automobile accident. She is conscious upon admission. A physical examination and x-rays reveal a transection of the spinal cord at T-4. The nurse should give the highest priority to which information?

1. The client has an allergy to iodine.
2. The client last voided seven hours ago.
3. The client smokes two packs of cigarettes a day.
4. The client is menstruating.

63. A 25-year-old female client is taking ampicillin (Amcill) and birth control pills containing estrogen. What information should the nurse provide?

1. Take both medications with breakfast to avoid gastric upset.
2. When used together, serum potassium levels may rise.
3. The effectiveness of the birth control pills may be reduced while the client is taking ampicillin.
4. Urticaria is much more common when antibiotics are given with other drugs.

64. A client, 65 years old, is admitted to the hospital for surgery after finding a lump in his right testicle. He asks the nurse, "Do you think the doctor will find cancer?" Which is the best nursing response initially?

1. "Most lumps found in the testicles are benign."
2. "It must be difficult for you not to know what the doctor will find."
3. "I think that you should discuss this with your doctor."
4. "It might be, but the doctor won't know until the surgery is performed."

65. A client's psychiatrist orders lithium four times daily. When administering medications on the sixth day, the nurse notes that the client's laboratory report indicates a serum lithium level of 1.0 mEq/liter. Based on this lab report, the most appropriate nursing action at this time is to:

1. Withhold the next dose of lithium and notify the psychiatrist.
2. Ask that the laboratory test be repeated.
3. Assess the client for possible toxic effects.
4. Administer the next dose of lithium as ordered.

66. A client is seen in the clinic in the 28th week of gestation. Her blood pressure is 160/100 and she has 2+ protein in her urine. She complains that all her shoes are too tight. Her doctor recommends hospitalization. The nurse who is admitting the client must select a bed for the new client. Each room on the unit is a semiprivate room. Which roommate should the nurse select for this client?

1. A 20-year-old primigravida who enjoys loud rock-and-roll music.
2. A 32-year-old multigravida who enjoys reading romance novels.
3. A 24-year-old C-section who watches soap operas and game shows on TV.
4. A 22-year-old primigravida who has many visitors during the afternoon and evening.

67. A client asks the nurse how relaxation techniques will help his gastric pain. "Can't I just take the Tagamet that my physician has prescribed?" In responding to his question, the nurse is guided by the knowledge that:

1. Gastric ulcer is a stress-related illness, and his stress levels and emotional issues are contributing to the exacerbation of his symptoms.
2. He is in denial, because he is refusing to acknowledge that stress is playing a role in the progress of his illness.
3. Gastric ulcer and other psychosomatic illnesses are caused by stress and can't be cured with only medical or surgical treatments.
4. The client is displaying the "typical ulcer personality" of a competitive, aggressive person who is defending against unresolved dependency needs.

68. A six-week-old infant with AIDS is being prepared for discharge. The child's primary caregiver is the grandmother. Which statement by the grandmother would alert the nurse to a need for further instruction?

1. "I know that handwashing is an important preventative measure."
2. "I'll use disposable diapers, discarding them in separate plastic bags."
3. "Blood spills should be washed up immediately with hot soapy water."
4. "Gloves should be worn by all persons changing the baby's diapers."

69. The most important nursing goal for a client who is admitted with an acute exacerbation of ulcerative colitis is:

1. To provide emotional support.
2. To prevent skin breakdown.
3. To maintain fluid and electrolyte balance.
4. To promote physical rest.

70. The nurse observes a 72-year-old client trying to climb over the side rails of the bed. The nurse is placing a vest restraint on the client when the daughter arrives and says to the nurse, "My mother does not need to be tied down in bed. I've been caring for her for years, and she hasn't fallen out of bed yet." The best initial response by the nurse is:

1. "I just saw your mother trying to climb over the side rails. Since I am concerned about her falling and hurting herself, I think this is best for her safety."
2. "Tell me how you managed to care for her at home."
3. "Hospital policy requires restraint vests on clients who are at risk for falling. I just saw your mother trying to climb over the rails. You don't want her to get hurt, do you?"
4. "The elderly may become confused in an unfamiliar place and do things they wouldn't do at home. It is difficult to see her restrained. While you are with her, the restraints can be off. Let me know when you are ready to leave."

71. The nurse is caring for a client who is recovering from surgery. He has a urinary catheter in place that needs to be irrigated. The correct approach to prevent injury to the mucosa of the bladder is:

1. Gently compress the ball of the syringe to instill the irrigating solution.
2. Quickly instill the irrigating solution, using some pressure to loosen any clots or mucous.
3. After instilling the solution, apply gentle pressure to remove the irrigating solution from the bladder.
4. Place a sterile cap on the end of the drainage tubing to protect it from contamination.

72. A 21-year-old client is admitted to the hospital because of extreme weight loss. It is noted on the admission assessment that the client believes that she is overweight at 88 pounds. What aspect of care should the nurse consider the first priority for this client's care?

1. Assessing the client's nutritional status.
2. Obtaining a psychiatric consult.
3. Planning a therapeutic diet for the client.
4. Talking to family members to find out more about the client's self-concept.

73. A client is hospitalized for a closed reduction of a fractured femur and application of a cast. A vital nursing action in the care of this client is to:

1. Perform neurovascular checks of the extremities.
2. Use the palms of the hands when moving an extremity with a wet cast.
3. Provide an instrument for the client to scratch the itching areas of skin under the cast.
4. Petal the edges of the cast to provide smooth edges.

74. After detoxification, a client begins the rehabilitation phase of treatment. He tells the nurse that he cannot imagine living his life without alcohol. The nurse's best response is based on what knowledge?

1. He will be more successful if he focuses on goals for short periods of time such as "today" or "this week".
2. He is likely to drink again when under stress.
3. He will not be successful if he is not strongly motivated.
4. He may require treatment with Antabuse to maintain sobriety.

75. While performing a vaginal exam on an obstetrical client, the nurse notes a glistening white cord in the vagina. The first nursing action is to:

1. Return to the nurses' station to place an emergency call to the physician.
2. Start oxygen at six to 10 liters, and assess the client's vital signs.
3. Cover the cord with a sterile moist saline dressing.
4. Apply manual pressure on the presenting part and have the mother get into a knee-chest position.

76. A client is in the hospital and has just found out that her mother died of a heart attack. She is crying and has her face buried in the pillow. The most therapeutic nursing response is to:

1. Return in fifteen minutes to see how the client is doing.
2. Sit with the client for a little while.
3. Tell the client that she will feel better in the morning.
4. Share with the client that the nurse's mother died within the last year and that the nurse knows just how she feels.

77. A client with asthma is receiving an oxygen concentration of 35%. The nurse knows that achievement of the therapeutic goal of this treatment is best demonstrated by:

1. Absence of adventitious breath sounds.
2. PaO2 92.
3. Heart rate increase of 25 beats/min.
4. Bicarbonate level of 25 mEq/liter.

78. The primary nurse learns that an obsessive-compulsive client has a full set of dentures because he eroded all his tooth enamel with his brushing rituals. He also brushes his tongue several times a day, and has developed several ulcerations on it. His nursing care plan should set which goal as the highest initial priority?

1. He will eliminate his brushing and mouth care rituals.
2. He will verbalize the underlying cause of his behavior.
3. He will seek out the nurse when he is feeling anxious.
4. He will reestablish healthy tissue in his mouth and tongue.

79. The nurse is informed during report that a post-operative client has not voided for eight hours. The initial nursing action is to:

1. Assist the client to the bathroom.
2. Place the client on a bed pan and pour warm water over her perineum.
3. Palpate and percuss the client's bladder.
4. Catheterize the client.

80. A three-year-old is being admitted with nephrotic syndrome. The best roommate the nurse can select for this client is:

1. A 16-year-old recovering postoperatively from a ruptured appendix.
2. An eight-year-old with leukemia.
3. Another toddler with rheumatic fever.
4. No roommate, isolation is required.

81. A client is to receive antibiotics. The priority nursing action when preparing to administer this medication is to:

1. Determine if the client has any allergies.
2. Determine the route of administration.
3. Check the client's name band.
4. Check the dosage against the physician's order.

82. Before administering lithium, the nurse checks the client's latest lab report for her serum lithium level. She notes a level of 1.2 mEq/L. What is the best action for the nurse to take next?

1. Administer the next prescribed dose of lithium.
2. Suggest the blood test be repeated.
3. Withhold the next dose of lithium and notify the psychiatrist of the lab results.
4. Ask the client how he is feeling, to identify any untoward effects.

83. A client is admitted to the psychiatric unit with a diagnosis of acute depression. After being hospitalized for a few weeks, the client says to the nurse, "I'm a terrible person, and I should be dead." Which response by the nurse is appropriate initially?

1. "That is why you are here. We are trying to help you with your bad feelings."
2. "Feeling that way must be awful. What makes you feel so terrible?"
3. "Feeling like a terrible person is part of your illness. As you get better, those feelings will lessen."
4. "You are not terrible. You are not a bad person."

84. The nurse in a long-term care facility finds an elderly client on the floor. After having the client examined by the physician, the most important nursing action is to:

1. Call the family to stay with the client.
2. Provide for the safety and protection of the client.
3. Apply wrist and leg restraints to prevent the client from falling out of bed.
4. Obtain an order for medication to sedate the client.

85. A 25-year-old man was admitted one week ago with a diagnosis of schizophrenia, paranoid type. Since his admission, he has had several verbal outbursts of anger but has not been violent. A staff member tells the nurse that the client is pacing up and down the hall very rapidly and muttering to himself in an angry manner. The best initial nursing action is to:

1. Prepare an intramuscular injection of haloperidol (Haldol) to give him p.r.n.
2. Observe the client's behavior and approach him in a non-threatening manner.
3. Gather several staff members and approach the client together.
4. Contact the client's psychiatrist and request an order to place him in seclusion.

86. Betamethasone (Celestone) is administered to a client at 30 weeks gestation to reduce the risk of RDS in the neonate. The infant is born after two injections are given. In planning nursing care for the infant, which finding should be anticipated as a result of the administration of betamethasone to the mother?

1. Rapid pulse rate.
2. Sternal retractions.
3. Hypoglycemia.
4. Hypothermia.

87. In preparing to begin an aminophylline infusion, which nursing approach would be best?

1. Prepare a solution containing enough drug to last 24 hours.
2. Obtain an infusion pump to regulate the flow of the drug.
3. Insert a large IV catheter to assure adequate dilution.
4. Initiate measurement of intake and output to detect fluid retention.

88. A client is being given an aminoglycoside for his bacterial infection. The nurse can aid in minimizing the risk of aminoglycoside toxicity by:

1. Weighing the client daily.
2. Encouraging the client to drink at least 2000 ml of fluids daily.
3. Monitoring blood pressure prior to drug administration.
4. Instructing the client to take the medicine with food.

89. A client is hospitalized for gastrointestinal bleeding and is being treated with temazepam (Restoril). After the client's physician examined him, the nurse noted the physician wrote an order for the client to begin taking amitriptyline (Elavil). Which action by the nurse would be best initially?

1. Revise his medication schedule so that the Elavil is administered during the day and the Restoril at bedtime.
2. Monitor the client's vital signs closely.
3. Question the physician about administering both Elavil and Restoril to the client.
4. Assess the client for signs and symptoms of depression.

90. The nurse is caring for a client with a myocardial infarction who is taking chlorothiazide (Diuril) and digoxin (Lanoxin). Which diet would be most appropriate to include in this client's nursing care?

1. Diet low in sodium and saturated fats, high in potassium.
2. Diet low in unsaturated fats, sodium, and potassium.
3. Diet high in potassium, Vitamin C, and protein.
4. Diet low in sodium and saturated and unsaturated fats.

91. The nurse is caring for a diabetic client who is currently taking cephalexin (Keflex). The nurse should advise the client that:

1. Clinitest or copper sulfate urine glucose tests give false positive results.
2. Blood sugar may drop without warning.
3. A source of sugar should always be carried with the client.
4. A medic alert bracelet should always be worn.

92. A client, age 82, is admitted to the psychiatric unit for a diagnostic work-up because she has become increasingly forgetful and disoriented at home. She has been taking lorazepam (Ativan) 0.5 mg p.r.n. to control her restlessness. In planning nursing care for this client, it would be unnecessary to include close observation for:

1. Orthostatic hypotension.
2. Increased anxiety.
3. Hyperexcitation.
4. Hallucinations.

93. A client with chronic emphysema is taking theophylline (Theo-dur) at home. During the home care nurse's visit, which statement by the client would warrant immediate action?

1. "I just lie awake at night, worrying about the medical bills."
2. "I must have the flu. I was vomiting all night."
3. "I don't have my usual appetite. Nothing tastes good to me."
4. "I feel better if I have a big glass of milk with my pill."

94. A client, age 22, is admitted with a diagnosis of acute psychotic reaction, rule out schizophrenia. Because the client is very agitated, he is started on chlorpromazine (Thorazine) 100 mg t.i.d. After three days, he is much calmer and his nurse begins to teach him about his medication. Which statement by the nurse is most appropriate?

1. "This medication is a sedative to calm you down."
2. "This medication acts on the chemical regulators in your brain to help control your symptoms."
3. "This medication will cure your disorder."
4. "We do not know how this medication works, but we do know it will help you control your behavior."

95. A client scheduled for surgery the next day to create an ileal conduit is receiving neomycin sulfate (Mycifradin Sulfate). What is the nurse's best explanation to the client for her receiving neomycin preoperatively?

1. To suppress of intestinal bacteria preoperatively, in order to decrease the risk of postoperative infection.
2. To decrease the number of pathogenic bacteria and decrease the number of loose stools.
3. To sterilize the bowel and prevent the risk of serious postoperative complications.
4. To prevent auditory impairment and nephrotoxicity during the postoperative period.

96. A client, age 22, is admitted with pneumocystis carinii pneumonitis. The physician prescribes sulfamethoxazole trimethoprim (Bactrim), and a Foley catheter is inserted to monitor urinary output. Which nursing intervention would be most effective in reducing the risk of crystalluria secondary to sulfonamide therapy?

1. Encouraging fluid intake to 3000 cc/24 hours.
2. Irrigating the Foley catheter with normal saline every eight hours.
3. Monitoring specific gravity of urine every eight hours.
4. Providing foods/fluids likely to maintain an acidic pH of the urine.

97. A client is to receive IM methylergonovine (Methergine). In caring for the client, the nurse knows that the administration of IM Methergine is contraindicated in which situation?

1. Boggy fundus one hour after vaginal delivery.
2. Large amount of vaginal bleeding following abortion at 16 weeks.
3. Client with history of previous postpartum hemorrhage in recovery room.
4. Client who has not delivered placenta 20 minutes following birth of baby.

98. A client is receiving propranolol (Inderal) for anxiety. In reviewing the client's discharge plans, the nurse needs to emphasize that:

1. Inderal should be discontinued by gradually tapering it off over time.
2. Inderal should not be taken during pregnancy.
3. Inderal is contraindicated for clients with asthma.
4. Inderal is a safe medication with no known adverse effects.

99. A 55-year-old client has been taking trifluoperazine (Stelazine) for five years to control her paranoid thoughts. When the client's brother comes to visit, he tells the nurse that he believes all psychiatric medications are a form of "chemical mind control." The nurse's best response to the brother will incorporate which information about antipsychotic medications?

1. They act directly on specific neurotransmitters in the brain to control the client's psychotic symptoms.
2. They act to sedate the client so she cannot engage in behavior that will cause difficulty for either herself or others.
3. They are a cure for psychotic disorders, like schizophrenic reactions, and are therefore an important part of his sister's treatment plan.
4. They have been in use for close to 30 years and are safe and effective drugs for clients who have problems like his sister's.

100. Which measure would the nurse select as providing the most accurate determination of renal impairment secondary to administration of amphotericin B (Fungizone)?

1. Intake and output.
2. Daily weights.
3. Serum creatinine levels.
4. Serial potassium levels.

CONGRATULATIONS! You have reached the end of the Final Exam. **Now, turn to Chapter Eleven to score your exam, assess your progress, and read the rationales.**

NOTES

Chapter 11

Answers and Analysis

Before you turn the page and look for the answers to the Final Exam, read the following reminders. And remember, the more test questions you answer during your review practice sessions, the better you will become at taking this kind of exam. Practice makes perfect!

Making the Most of Your Final Exam Results

❶ If you answered a question incorrectly, **determine whether you did not know the material or just misread the question.** If you misread a question, identify the **critical element** that was overlooked. You need to minimize the questions you are answering incorrectly because of misreading!

❷ When you review the answers to the questions -- using either this chapter or the Answers and Analysis post-test section on the diskette -- be sure to read the rationales: You might have answered a question correctly using an incorrect rationale! (In your practice sessions, always review the rationales.)

❸ Try to determine how many questions you answered correctly **by using one of the three test-taking strategies.** When you are unsure of an answer, eliminating incorrect options and using test-taking strategies can increase your score dramatically!

❹ Use the Assessment Scale on the following page to assess your progress.

Assessment Scale	
Score	**Recommendation**
Less than 65%	OOPS! Don't get discouraged! Spend some time reviewing the basic concepts and strategies in Chapters 3 and 4, and try again.
65-75% and	Good work. Try reviewing the Test-Taking Tips" "Points to Remember," and keep practicing.
75-85%	Very good. You are becoming a good strategist! Keep answering practice questions until the exam.
85%+	Superior work!! Continue to apply these principles, and try to ace the exam!

❺ After calculating your score and analyzing your answers, you should **continue to practice answering questions and assessing your progress on a daily basis.** This is especially important for NCLEX candidates! But nursing students should continue to practice these new test-taking skills, too.

❻ If you are an NCLEX candidate and were not able to use the computer diskette enclosed with this book, be sure to plan some time on a computer in your learning lab to practice taking a computerized exam. You might also wish to use some of the other NCLEX review materials, including comprehensive review manuals, audio or video tapes, and especially Q&A books. MEDS, Inc. also offers comprehensive Q&A review software, which uses the same Personalized Performance Analysis as the diskette accompanying this book. The more test questions you answer, the better!

We hope *Successful Problem-Solving and Test-Taking* has revolutionized your approach to taking an exam, and to studying and reviewing material. You have acquired an important new professional skill.

GOOD LUCK IN YOUR COURSES, AND ON THE NCLEX!

1. **The nurse visits a client at home one week following his discharge after a myocardial infarction. He is taking chlorothiazide (Diuril) 500 mg daily and digoxin (Lanoxin) 0.25 mg daily. The nurse should give top priority to assessing the client's knowledge related to:**

    1. Sources of potassium.
    2. Sources of sodium.
    3. Activity restrictions.
    4. Signs of a heart attack.

    1. ***Very good! Because the client is taking both Diuril and digoxin, the nurse should focus on his knowledge related to sources of potassium. Diuril depletes potassium. If the potassium level is too low, digoxin toxicity may lead to serious cardiac arrhythmias. This is the top priority because lack of understanding may become life-threatening very quickly.***

    2. Wrong choice. The client is probably on a sodium restricted diet. Too much sodium will increase the cardiac workload. The nurse should assess the client's knowledge of sources of sodium but, based on the information provided in the case scenario, this is not the top priority.

    3. Wrong choice. The client will increase his activity gradually as he recuperates from the myocardial infarction. The nurse should assess the client's knowledge of activity restrictions but, based on the information provided in the case scenario, this is not the top priority.

    4. Wrong choice. The nurse should assess the client's knowledge of the signs of another heart attack but, based on the information provided in the case scenario, this is not the top priority.

2. **A adolescent client is to have a water system heating device ("K-Pad"), applied to a pulled muscle. The client tells the nurse that the device does not feel very warm. The most appropriate nursing action is to:**

    1. Tell the client that these heating devices never feel hot.
    2. Check the temperature setting on the heating unit and feel the pad for warmth.
    3. Call the appropriate repair department and have them fix the unit.
    4. Turn the temperature up on the unit if it doesn't feel warm enough to the client.

    1. Wrong. Although these heating units do feel warm and not hot, the unit may not be at a therapeutic temperature, and should be assessed to see if it is working properly.

    2. Correct! The nurse should check that the device is set to the temperature recommended by the manufacturer. The nurse should also assess whether the pad feels warm.

    3. Incorrect! The unit may not be malfunctioning. It should be assessed by the nurse before any other action is taken. If the unit is malfunctioning, it should be replaced with another unit, and the malfunctioning unit should be sent to the repair department.

    4. Incorrect! The temperature should not be set above the recommended setting, to avoid causing a burn to the client.

3. **A 34-year-old client who weighs 288 pounds says to the nurse, "I'm going to have surgery and have my stomach stapled in order to lose weight. I've tried everything else, and nothing seems to work." Which response by the nurse would be therapeutic?**

    1. "That's a pretty drastic measure. Are you sure that is what you want to do?"
    2. "I hear that the surgery is only a temporary measure, and if you have the staples removed you will only gain the weight back again."
    3. "It must be difficult to be overweight and not able to lose weight. What does your husband think about the surgery?"
    4. "Can you tell me about the possible consequences and side effects of this type of surgery?"

    1. Incorrect. This response by the nurse is judgmental and questions the decision made by the client. There is no encouragement from the nurse that promotes further communication from the client. This is not a therapeutic nursing response.

    2. Incorrect. This may or may not be an accurate statement, but it does not promote therapeutic communication. The client is frustrated about her weight and needs to express her feelings. This response indicates to the client that her situation is hopeless.

    3. This response is only half correct. The first part uses the therapeutic communication tool of empathy, but the second part (asking about the husband's feelings) blocks communication by focusing on an inappropriate person. Starting an incorrect answer off with correct buzzwords is a common ploy in distractors, which is why memorization alone is worthless for the NCLEX. Recognizing buzzwords without understanding the theory behind them and its proper application can lead the nurse candidate to choose distractors like this one.

    4. Congratulations! This response asks for clarification of the client's understanding of the surgery and promotes further communication.

> ***TEST-TAKING TIP:*** *This is an implementation question that asks for an appropriate response by the nurse. In communication questions, look for an option that uses a therapeutic communication tool and addresses the client's feelings and concerns.*

4. **The nurse finds an elderly client standing in a puddle of water in the hallway of the unit. The nurse does not know this client. What should the nurse do first?**

1. Ask the client for her name and room number.
2. Wipe up the water until the floor is completely dry.
3. Call the supervisor for assistance in identifying the client.
4. Have the client wait in the lounge until security arrives.

1. *Incorrect. The issue in this question is the puddle of water on the floor. The water on the floor threatens the safety of the client and others on the unit. After eliminating the safety hazard, the nurse can identify the client and assist with getting her back to where she belongs.*
2. ***Very good! The issue in this question is the puddle of water on the floor. The water on the floor threatens the safety of the client and others on the unit. The nurse's first action should be to alleviate the safety hazard by wiping up the water. Maslow's Hierarchy of Needs indicates that, when no physiological need exists, safety needs should receive priority.***

> ***TEST-TAKING TIP:*** *The idea of water on the floor is repeated in this option. The test-taking strategy of looking for similar words or phrases in the question would identify this option as a possible answer if you were unsure of the best response.*

3. *Wrong! The issue in this question is the puddle of water on the floor. The water on the floor threatens the safety of the client and others on the unit. After eliminating the safety hazard, the nurse can identify the client and assist with getting her back to where she belongs.*
4. *The issue in this question is the puddle of water on the floor. The water on the floor threatens the safety of the client and others on the unit. Asking the client to wait in the lounge until security arrives does not assure safety. Someone may still slip on the puddle of water and injure themselves.*

5. **The nurse caring for a client on the evening before his scheduled left below-the-knee amputation provides preoperative teaching, including deep breathing and coughing. Which question would be most helpful for the nurse to ask the client, to evaluate the effectiveness of the preoperative teaching?**

1. "Do you understand what we have just discussed about deep breathing and coughing?"
2. "Do you think that you will need to have a sedative to help you sleep tonight?"
3. "Will you demonstrate for me the correct method of deep breathing and coughing?"
4. "Do you have any questions concerning your scheduled surgical procedure?"

1. *Not the best option! This question asks the client about the content of the preoperative teaching in the form of a closed question, which requires only a "yes" or "no" answer. The client could answer "yes" regardless of the true state of his understanding. This is not the best question to ask.*
2. *Wrong choice. The test question asked you to select a question that the nurse should ask to evaluate preoperative teaching. In this option, the nurse is asking about the need for a sedative, not about the client's understanding of preoperative teaching. Although the question is an appropriate question for the nurse to ask at this time, it is not the correct answer because it does not relate to the issue in the question.*
3. ***Excellent! This question asks the client about the content of the preoperative teaching. In addition, the question requests a return demonstration of deep breathing and coughing. If the preoperative teaching has been effective, the client will be able to do the return demonstration. If additional teaching is required, the client will be unable to do the return demonstration properly. This is the best question for evaluating the effectiveness of preoperative teaching.***
4. *Wrong choice. This question is an appropriate question for the nurse to ask at this time. It is not the correct answer, however, because the stem of this test question asks you to select a question that the nurse should ask to evaluate preoperative teaching. Here, the nurse is asking about the client's understanding of the surgical procedure. The client's questions concerning the surgical procedure should be referred to the doctor.*

6. **The nurse is conducting a preoperative interview three days prior to admitting a seven-year-old female for tonsillectomy. The child's mother requests information to prepare her daughter for hospitalization. The nurse knows that the child was hospitalized last year for a fractured femur. Which nursing actions would best meet this child's needs for preparation?**

1. Suggest a role play, and provide materials.
2. Remind the child of the experience of her past hospitalization.
3. Read the child a story about another child having a similar operation.
4. Tell the child she is only going in to have her throat checked.

1. ***Yes, concrete experiences are the most meaningful learning for the school age child. This is the rationale for pediatric orientation programs. Even if there is inadequate time for her***

to participate in such a program, a shortened version where she could practice with a mask and other equipment in a non-threatening environment would be helpful.

2. *No, be careful! Past experiences, especially traumatic ones, may not have been positive.*
3. *No, this isn't the best response. This is somewhat abstract, and abstract thinking is not highly developed in the seven-year-old child.*
4. *Wrong! Never lie to a child. This is inappropriate under any circumstances.*

7. A client is admitted to the hospital in respiratory distress. The doctor orders oxygen via mask and the client to be placed in Fowler's position. Which nursing action is most important for this client at this time?

1. Support and align the hands with the forearms.
2. Use handrolls.
3. Raise the head of the bed to allow for greater lung expansion.
4. Support the feet at right angles to the lower legs.

1. *Wrong choice. This option does not address the issue of the question, which is a nursing action to counter respiratory distress. Supporting and aligning the hands prevents potential contractures of the wrist. Try again.*
2. *Wrong choice. This option does not address the issue of the question, which is a nursing action to counter respiratory distress. Handrolls aid in preventing contractures by maintaining the fingers and thumbs in a functional position. Try again.*
3. ***Good! The elevation of the head of the bed allows for greater lung expansion and decreased respiratory effort. This option correctly addresses the issue of the question, which is a nursing action to counter respiratory distress.***

> ***TEST-TAKING TIP:*** *The similar words "respiratory" and "lung expansion" are found in the question and this option, respectively. The test-taking strategy of looking for similar words or phrases in the question would identify this option as a possible answer if you were unsure of the best response.*

4. *Wrong choice. This option does not address the issue of the question, which is a nursing action to counter respiratory distress. Supporting the feet prevents foot drop and contractures at the ankle. Try again.*

8. A 23-year-old gravida 1, para 0 is admitted to the hospital at 38 weeks gestation with pregnancy induced hypertension. Which finding would the nurse identify as inconsistent with the admitting diagnosis?

1. 3+ protein in the urine.
2. Deep tendon reflexes of +1.
3. Blood pressure of 148/98.
4. 1+ pitting sacral edema.

1. *Wrong choice. Symptoms of pregnancy induced hypertension include proteinuria, edema, and elevated blood pressure. A finding of 3+ protein in the urine would be consistent with the diagnosis of pregnancy induced hypertension. This question has a false response stem, so the correct answer is something that the nurse would NOT expect to find in an assessment of the client.*
2. ***Good! In pregnancy induced hypertension, the nurse would expect to find an increased deep tendon reflex, not a decreased deep tendon reflex.***

> ***TEST-TAKING TIP:*** *Because this question has a false response stem, the correct answer is something the nurse would NOT expect to find in an assessment of the client.*

3. *Wrong choice. This would be consistent with the admitting diagnosis. Symptoms of pregnancy induced hypertension include proteinuria, edema, and elevated blood pressure. Blood pressure of 148/98 is elevated and would be consistent with the diagnosis of pregnancy induced hypertension. The correct answer is something the nurse would NOT expect to find in an assessment of the client.*
4. *Wrong choice. This would be consistent with the admitting diagnosis. Symptoms of pregnancy induced hypertension include edema, proteinuria, and elevated blood pressure. A finding of 1+ pitting sacral edema would be consistent with the diagnosis of pregnancy induced hypertension. The correct answer is something the nurse would NOT expect to find in an assessment of the client.*

9. When the nurse enters a client's room, the client's son tells the nurse, "You people can't do anything right. Ever since my father was admitted to this hospital, it has been one mistake after another. I am taking him out of here before you kill him." The nurse's most helpful response to the son is:

1. "You feel that your father is not being well cared for?"
2. "We have the best intentions for the clients."
3. "I'll get the supervisor for you."
4. "Your father hasn't complained about the care. What specifically is the problem?"

1. ***Excellent! This response uses the communication tool of restatement and focuses on the issue. This response encourages the son to express his concerns to the nurse. The nurse needs more information from the client before problem-solving can occur. This response also focuses on the "here and now."***
2. *Incorrect. This response is a defensive remark by the nurse, which is a communication block.*

This response implies that whatever is bothering the son cannot be valid, and this response may escalate the situation. A therapeutic response would encourage the son to tell the nurse why he feels upset concerning his father's care.

3. *Incorrect. The son is the client in this communication question. This response puts the client's feelings on hold by asking him to wait until the supervisor arrives. Therapeutic communication addresses the "here and now," and does not "pass the buck" to another person. Indeed, the supervisor may become involved, but the best response by the nurse is to address the client's immediate needs.*
4. *Incorrect. The son is the client in this communication question. This response focuses on the father, but the son is the one who has voiced concerns to the nurse. This response implies that the son's feelings cannot be valid since his father has not voiced any complaints. This devalues the client's feelings. This response is not therapeutic.*

10. After a myocardial infarction, which vital signs assessment should the nurse recognize as possible indications of cardiogenic shock?

1. BP - 180/100, P - 90, irregular.
2. BP - 130/80, P - 100 regular.
3. BP - 90/50, P - 50 regular.
4. BP - 80/60, P - 110, irregular.

1. *Incorrect. These vital signs are not seen in a shock-like state. Choose again.*
2. *No, these vital signs are within normal limits. Recall the pathophysiology of shock, and make a more appropriate selection.*
3. *This is only partially correct. The client in cardiogenic shock will be hypotensive, but will not be bradycardic. Choose another option.*
4. ***Good analysis! The classic signs of cardiogenic shock are low blood pressure, rapid and weak pulse, cold, clammy skin, decreased urinary output, and cerebral hypoxia.***

11. An 18-year-old client is hospitalized for treatment of severe depression. Which nursing approach should be included in the plan of care for this client?

1. Giving the client choices.
2. Spending time with the client.
3. Providing a chess game.
4. Encouraging decision-making.

1. *Incorrect. Making choices is difficult for a depressed client.*

> ***TEST-TAKING TIP:*** *Note that this option is very similar to Option 4. Neither one can be correct! Such similar options should be eliminated.*

2. ***Correct. Because depressed clients frequently have suicidal tendencies, spending time with the client will provide for her safety. Depression also involves diminished self-esteem, and spending time with the client conveys to her that she is worth the nurse's time and attention. This action is therapeutic for the client and provides for her safety.***
3. *Try again. An intellectual game such as chess would not be a good activity for a depressed client. Non-intellectual activities such as latch hook or needle work would be a better choice. Read all of the other options, and then try to select the best one.*
4. *Try again. Decision-making is difficult for a depressed client.*

> ***TEST-TAKING TIP:*** *Note that this option is very similar to Option 1. Neither one can be correct! Such similar options should be eliminated.*

12. A two-year-old is hospitalized with bacterial pneumonia. The nurse will monitor her respiratory status closely. Which signs/symptoms would the nurse identify as the earliest indication of respiratory difficulty?

1. Respiratory rate of 40 to 48.
2. Blood pressure of 80/60.
3. Cyanosis of mucous membranes.
4. Circumoral/periorbital pallor.

1. ***Good choice! One early indication of respiratory difficulty is an increased respiratory rate. A respiratory rate of 40 to 48 is rapid for a two-year-old.***
2. *Incorrect. A blood pressure of 80/60 is within normal limits for a two-year-old and does not indicate increased respiratory difficulty.*
3. *Wrong choice. Cyanosis of mucous membranes is certainly a sign of respiratory difficulty, but it is a late sign. The nurse should be alert for early signs so that appropriate intervention can begin. Try again.*
4. *Incorrect. Circumoral/periorbital pallor is certainly a sign of respiratory difficulty. However, this is a late sign. The nurse should be alert for early signs so that appropriate intervention can begin.*

13. A client is in labor and is admitted with a blood pressure of 86/52. She is four centimeters dilated and uncomfortable. The nurse should give immediate consideration to which nursing action?

1. Call the physician to report the blood pressure.
2. Turn the client on her side and retake her blood pressure.
3. Reassure the client that everything is all right.
4. Ask the client if she would like some pain medication.

1. *Wrong! The need for adequate blood pressure is a physiological need that requires immediate intervention. Try to identify another option that addresses this need.*
2. ***Good choice! Supine hypotension is a frequent cause of low blood pressure in pregnant clients. By turning the client on her side and retaking the blood pressure, the nurse is attempting to correct the low blood pressure and then reassessing. The need for adequate blood pressure is a physiological need that requires immediate intervention.***
3. *Incorrect. Reassuring the client that everything is all right is not a priority action and may be false reassurance. Maslow's Hierarchy of Needs indicates that physiological needs should receive priority.*
4. *Wrong choice. The issue in this question is labor and low blood pressure. The need for adequate blood pressure is a physiological need that requires immediate intervention. This option is focused on the client's discomfort, which is not life-threatening and may not require medication once other comfort measures can be instituted. The client's comfort should be addressed as soon as the nurse has determined that the blood pressure is stable.*

14. During a client's postoperative recovery from an ileostomy, the nurse begins teaching her stoma care. The client refuses to look at her ostomy and tells the nurse, "I'd rather be dead than have to live with this all my life." The appropriate nursing response is:

1. "I can't imagine what you must be feeling; it must be awful."
2. "I'll call your physician and see if something can be ordered to help you to relax."
3. "There's no reason to feel like that. Things will get better."
4. "You appear upset. Would you like to talk?"

1. *This response may appear empathetic, but it is excessive and is not therapeutic. Expressing excessive approval can be as harmful to the nurse/client relationship as stating disapproval.*
2. *No, this response ignores the client's statement and changes the subject, which conveys a lack of empathy. This response does not encourage the client to express her feelings.*
3. *No, this offers false reassurance to the client, which is a block to therapeutic communication.*
4. ***Good choice. This response uses the therapeutic communication tool of empathy, and in a nonthreatening manner encourages the client to verbalize her feelings. It conveys to the client a caring attitude and a willingness to listen.***

15. A client was hospitalized for major depression and treated with nortriptyline (Pamelor). As the client is preparing for discharge, which statement by the client would indicate to the nurse that she needs further instruction?

1. "I'm glad this medicine helps me. My husband and I would like to start our family as soon as possible."
2. "If I should feel hopeless and suicidal again, I have the telephone number of my therapist to call for help."
3. "I hope I will not have to continue taking medicine forever. I guess I'll have to see how I do."
4. "I plan to see my psychiatrist regularly. She told me if I continue to do well, I can probably stop taking my medication in nine to 12 months."

1. ***Correct choice. This statement indicates that the client needs further instruction. Tricyclic antidepressants should be avoided during pregnancy, especially during the first trimester, because they are associated with fetal anomalies.***
2. *Wrong choice. This statement by the client does not indicate that the client needs further instruction. Since 60% of depressed persons experience suicidal thoughts, each hospitalized client should have a plan for obtaining help if these thoughts recur after discharge. The client's statement indicates that she has a good plan to follow, which the nurse should reinforce. The stem asks for the statement that indicates a knowledge deficit. Identify another option.*
3. *Wrong choice. This is a realistic statement. It does not indicate a need for further instruction. An estimated 15% of clients with depressive illness develop chronic or recurring symptoms of depression. Clients should remain under the care of a mental health professional after hospital discharge so their condition can be monitored. The stem in this question asks for the statement that indicates a knowledge deficit. Identify another option.*
4. *Wrong choice. This statement by the client is appropriate. Most clients remain on their antidepressant for nine to 12 months after recovering from an episode of depression. A rebound depression can occur if the medication is discontinued too soon. This statement by the client does not indicate a need for further instruction. The stem in this question asks for the statement that indicates a knowledge deficit. Try again.*

16. A 22-year-old client has had surgery on his foot and has just been returned to his room from the recovery room. The initial assessment indicates that he is stable. An hour later, his roommate turns on the call light and tells the nurse that the client has gotten up and hopped on one foot to the bathroom, using his IV pole for support. Which action should the nurse take initially to provide for the client's safety?

1. Open the bathroom door to assess if the client is okay.
2. Assist the client in ambulating back to bed and get him a urinal.
3. Explain to the client that it is not safe for him to be hopping around on one foot.
4. Get a wheelchair and help the client back to bed when he is done in the bathroom.

1. This action is inappropriate. Even though the client should not have hopped to the bathroom, the nurse should respect his privacy and knock on the door to determine if he is okay.

2. Wrong. The client will have to hop back to bed with the nurse helping to support him, which is not a very stable method of ambulation. This is not safe.

3. This is not the priority action. Since the client is already in the bathroom, getting the client safely back to bed is the priority issue for the nurse.

4. Good choice. Since the client is already in the bathroom, allow him to void, and then return him to his bed safely in a wheelchair. This is an implementation question, and the stem asks you to prioritize the actions. This option meets the physiological and safety needs of the client, while also respecting his privacy.

17. A 77-year-old client was hospitalized for observation after a fall that he experienced when he was walking for exercise. He is to ambulate for the first time since his fall. He tells the nurse that he is afraid to get up. The best response by the nurse is:

1. "There is nothing to be afraid of. The order wouldn't have been written if your doctor didn't think that you were ready."
2. "Tell me what concerns you about getting up today."
3. "I will have another person here to help you when you get up."
4. "Are you afraid of falling again?"

1. Wrong choice. This response does not facilitate a response from the client. It devalues his concerns by making the doctor's orders seem more important. It also focuses on the doctor and not on the client. A therapeutic response focuses on the client's feelings.

2. Excellent! This nursing response focuses on the client's feelings, and it gives value to the client's statement by directly addressing the client's concerns. This response uses the therapeutic communication tool of clarification and encourages the client to express to the nurse what he is feeling concerning ambulating.

3. Incorrect. This response may not address the client's concerns, since the nurse does not know why the client is afraid. Clarification is necessary before the nurse can plan to meet the client's needs. This response focuses on the nurse's action, and not on the client's feelings.

4. Incorrect. The nurse does not know why the client is afraid, but this is not the best clarification question to ask because it can be answered with a simple yes or no answer. The nurse should encourage the client to express his feelings. Try again.

18. To safely assess for correct placement of a nasogastric tube, the nurse should:

1. Instill 30 ml of saline to assess client tolerance.
2. Instill 10 ml of air into the tube and listen for gurgling sounds with a stethoscope over the gastric area.
3. Aspirate stomach contents with a syringe.
4. Place the end of the tube in water to assess for bubbling.

1. No! This procedure could be dangerous if the tube was incorrectly positioned in the lungs. Select a safer action.

2. Incorrect. This method does not provide for a sufficient amount of air to reach the stomach and make any gurgling sounds. At least 30 ml of air is needed for this test. There is a safer and more reliable method among the options given. Try again.

3. Correct. Placement should be checked by aspirating gastric contents with a syringe and testing the pH of the aspirate.

4. Never, never! This could be dangerous to the client if the tube was incorrectly positioned in the lungs, because the client could aspirate the water in the glass. Select a safer, more reliable option.

19. A psychiatric client is re-hospitalized after discontinuing her medication of her own accord. She has responded well to the support of the nurse-client relationship. The client's discharge plans include living with her parents and attending a job training program during the day. What is the most important goal for her remaining sessions with the nurse?

1. Reinforce the importance of taking her medications as prescribed.
2. Anticipate future problems and how she might handle them.
3. Terminate the nurse-client relationship.
4. Promote the client's self-confidence.

1. Incorrect. Reinforcing her medication regime is an important component of discharge planning, especially for this client, who had to be rehospitalized because she had stopped taking her medications. It is not the most important goal at this time. There is a better option.

2. This is an important component of discharge planning, but it is not the most important goal at this time.

3. ***Correct. The nurse should focus on ending their relationship by exploring the client's responses to the separation and dealing with any feelings of rejection that the client may have. This is the most important goal at this time, as it greatly affects the client's ability to establish positive relationships with health care providers in the future.***
4. *Promoting self-confidence is usually a component of the nursing care plan, but it is not the most important goal at this time.*

20. The nurse knows that the discharge teaching is successful for a client with Hepatitis A virus if the client indicates that she will never:

1. Donate blood.
2. Eat fried foods.
3. Vacation in a foreign country.
4. Order a salad in a restaurant.

1. ***Correct. Once a person has been infected with Hepatitis A virus, they can never donate blood.***
2. *Wrong choice. The client should not need to avoid fried foods permanently. Dietary fat is not contraindicated, but it may not be well tolerated. After the client recovers, she should be able to tolerate fats within two months.*
3. *Wrong choice. It is not necessary for the client to refrain from vacationing abroad. This in itself has no direct correlation to Hepatitis A virus.*
4. *Wrong choice. The client's fear is real if the initial cause of Hepatitis A was from eating at a restaurant. It is not necessary for the client to refrain from eating in restaurants, or from ordering salads, however, since this in itself has no direct correlation to Hepatitis A virus.*

21. A 55-year-old client is hospitalized following myocardial infarction. When transferring the client from a cart to his bed, the priority nursing action is to:

1. Have the client place his arms on his chest.
2. Lock the wheels on the cart and the bed.
3. Have at least four people to help with the transfer.
4. Use a draw sheet to move the client.

1. *Wrong choice. Although placing the arms across the chest helps protect the arms from injury, this option is not the priority action that is requested by the stem of the question. Make another choice.*
2. ***Right! Good prioritizing! Locking the wheels prevents the card or bed from moving apart or away from the client, and thus prevents the client from falling to the floor. This is the priority action for transferring a client.***
3. *Incorrect. Four people may or may not be the number needed for a transfer. The number will depend on the size of the client and the size of the persons performing the transfer. The case scenario does not provide enough information to establish this number of staff as necessary for the transfer.*
4. *Wrong choice. A draw sheet is often used to transfer clients between two level horizontal surfaces; however, this is neither a requirement nor a priority action. Try again.*

22. The nurse understands that which statement about reality testing is inaccurate?

1. It is an ego function.
2. It is impaired in psychotic individuals.
3. It is impaired in persons who are mentally retarded.
4. It is the capacity to distinguish thoughts, feelings, fantasies, and other experiences that originate inside the individual from those that are part of the outside environment.

1. *Wrong choice. This statement is accurate. Reality testing is an important ego function. Reality testing refers to the capacity to distinguish inner experiences from those that occur in the environment, and the capacity to establish intact ego boundaries. The stem of the question asks you to select an INACCURATE statement about reality testing. Try again.*
2. *Wrong choice. This statement is accurate. Reality testing is impaired in psychotic individuals. In psychotic disorders, the individual can no longer tell whether his or her own thoughts and feelings come from within, but instead may experience them as hallucinations and delusions originating from elsewhere. The stem of the question asks you to select an INACCURATE statement about reality testing. Try again.*
3. ***Correct choice. Reality testing is NOT impaired in persons who are mentally retarded, unless they are also psychotic. This is the INACCURATE statement sought in this test question.***
4. *Wrong choice. This is an accurate statement about reality testing. It is not the correct option in this question because the stem of the question asks you to select an option that is INACCURATE.*

23. The client is to receive a medication for control of tachycardia and an irregular heart rate. The nurse obtains the following vital signs prior to administering this medication: blood pressure 98/54, pulse 48, respirations 30, and temperature 98° F. The client's skin is cool, with cyanosis of the fingers and lips. The appropriate nursing action is to:

1. Administer the medication as ordered by the physician.
2. Omit the medication for a day or two, depending on the client's response and symptoms.

3. Notify the physician concerning the client's status before administering the medication.
4. Give the client one half of the ordered dose.

1. Wrong! Administering a medication that decreases the heart rate of a client with a pulse of 48 is unsafe, since the pulse rate may decrease even further. A pulse rate of 48 does not fall within the normal range, and results in a physiological need for oxygen for this client. Make another choice.

2. Sorry, this option is not the best choice. A pulse rate of 48 results in a physiological need for oxygen for this client. Withholding the medication is a possible nursing action, since the result of this action may be an increase in pulse rate. However, withholding the medication alone does not address all of the physiological needs identified in the case scenario. Be sure to read all the options before selecting the best one!

3. Very good! The assessment data gathered by the nurse indicates that the client is exhibiting signs and symptoms that are not within the normal parameters. A pulse rate of 48 results in a physiological need for oxygen for this client. Withholding the medication until the physician has been notified addresses the immediate physiological need of the client. The information needs to be communicated to the physician, who will determine which medical interventions are necessary.

4. Wrong. Changing or altering an ordered medication is a medical intervention, not a nursing action! Make another choice.

24. The nurse is preparing a teaching plan for a client being discharged following major abdominal surgery. The client will be doing her own dressing changes at home. Which technique is the most important for the nurse to include in the discharge teaching plan?

1. Opening bandages properly to maintain their sterility.
2. Maintaining strict aseptic technique.
3. Proper gloving technique.
4. Good handwashing technique.

1. Incorrect. The client is at risk for the transmission of microorganisms that may cause infection. The nurse should instruct the client in the proper method of opening bandages and other measures to prevent infection while changing the dressing. The home environment does not lend itself to the practice of aseptic technique, however, so the nurse must help the client improvise with the resources available. What is the most important action in preventing the spread of infection?

2. Incorrect. The client is at risk for the transmission of microorganisms that may cause an infection. The home environment does not lend itself to the practice of aseptic technique, however, so the nurse must help the client improvise with the resources available. What is the most important action in preventing the spread of infection?

3. Incorrect. The client is at risk for the transmission of microorganisms that may cause an infection. The home environment does not lend itself to the practice of aseptic technique, however, so the nurse must help the client improvise with the resources available. What is the most important action in preventing the spread of infection?

4. Correct! The client is at risk for the transmission of microorganisms that may cause an infection. The home environment may not lend itself to the entire practice of aseptic technique, so the nurse must help the client improvise with the resources available. Handwashing is the most important and most basic technique in preventing and controlling the transmission of pathogens and it should be practiced in every case.

25. A premature infant weighed only three pounds and seven ounces at birth. Following a lengthy stay in the hospital, her weight has increased to five pounds. She will be discharged soon. Which statement by the mother would indicate to the nurse that additional teaching is needed?

1. "My baby is so fragile that I will need to be very careful about everything that I do for her."
2. "I know that my baby will need to see the doctor regularly for awhile, and I have the appointments on my calendar."
3. "My mother is going to stay with me for several weeks to help me with my older children."
4. "I have the nursery, clothing, bottles, and diapers all ready for the day we bring our baby home."

1. Correct. Caring for a premature infant at home should not be any different from caring for a full term baby. This statement does reflect a need for further instruction.

2. Wrong choice. This statement by the client is appropriate and does not reflect a need for more instruction. Regular doctor appointments are especially important for premature infants because there is a greater risk for anemia and failure to thrive. You are looking for a statement by the mother that indicates a knowledge deficit.

3. Wrong choice. Extra help with household chores and older children is additional support which is helpful when mother and baby are adjusting to a new schedule. This statement by the client is appropriate. You are looking for a statement by the mother that indicates a knowledge deficit.

4. Wrong choice. This comment indicates that the mother is prepared to provide care for the baby at home. You are looking for a statement by the mother that indicates a knowledge deficit.

26. A client was told by her doctor that a lump was found in her breast and that a biopsy would have to be done. The client asks the nurse, "Do you think it is cancer?" Which nursing response is best initially?

1. "You seem to be worried about what the doctor may find."
2. "Do you have a family history of breast cancer?"
3. "We won't know anything until the biopsy is done."
4. "Most lumps are not cancerous, so you really shouldn't worry."

1. ***Good therapeutic response! Communication theory states that the nurse should focus on the client's feelings. This response focuses on her feelings of concern that she may have cancer. This response addresses the "here and now," using the therapeutic communication tools of empathy and clarification.***
2. This response is not therapeutic for this worried client. The response focuses on the client's family history, not on the client's feelings. The stem of the question asks which response is "best initially." After the client's feelings are addressed, information may be obtained in order to provide data concerning the incidence of breast cancer in families.
3. This response is not therapeutic. The response does not answer the client's question or promote further expression of the client's feelings. It blocks communication by putting the client's feelings of fear on hold.
4. This response is not therapeutic. The response offers false assurance and does not encourage the client to express her feelings concerning the fear of cancer. Saying "Don't worry" devalues the client's feelings.

27. A client has been told by the doctor that he has cancer and that it has advanced so far that treatment will not help. When the nurse enters the room to set up his bath equipment, he says to the nurse, "I'm not an invalid, you know. I can take care of myself. Get out and leave me alone." What is the best nursing response?

1. "I know that you are not an invalid. I was just trying to help you."
2. "It sounds to me like you are angry about something. Did somebody do something wrong?"
3. "You are pretty upset. Let's talk about it."
4. "I'll just set up this equipment for you to bathe and come back later when you're not so angry."

1. This is an incorrect option because this response focuses on the nurse and not on the client.
2. This option incorrectly assumes that the client is angry, and it focuses on inappropriate persons and issues. By asking if "somebody" did something wrong, it focuses on "somebody" else, instead of focusing on the client's feelings.
3. ***Good choice. This response addresses the emotional state of the client by stating that he is upset. The communication tool of clarification is used to promote therapeutic communication, which focuses first on the client's feelings.***
4. Incorrect. This option does not promote any communication with the client. It implies that his behavior is inappropriate and that the nurse is not willing to deal with it.

28. A six-year-old male is admitted with a spiral fracture of the humerus and multiple bruises of the forearm. The physician states that the injuries and other signs are suspicious for abuse. The nurse's initial goal is to:

1. Prevent further abuse of the client.
2. Encourage the client to express his feelings.
3. Determine who is responsible for the abuse.
4. Teach the parents the appropriate methods of discipline.

1. ***Very good! Safety first, then interventions that will decrease the chances of further abuse, such as education of parents.***
2. This is not the nurse's initial goal. You've missed the most important nursing responsibility to the client.

> ***TEST-TAKING TIP:*** *Use Maslow's Hierarchy of Needs to prioritize the nurse's actions.*

3. No, this is not the nurse's main responsibility.
4. No, you skipped an important issue and went right for teaching. Be careful; think about the basics that your 101 instructor taught you! Try again, using Maslow's Hierarchy of Needs to prioritize the nurse's actions.

29. While caring for a client, the nurse should practice good body mechanics and avoid muscle strain. In using good body mechanics, the nurse would avoid:

1. Moving muscles quickly, using short tugs.
2. Using the longest and strongest muscles of the body.
3. Leaning toward objects being pushed, such as a stretcher.
4. Carrying objects close to the body without touching your clothing.

1. ***You are right. This action is incorrect and should be avoided. Jerky movements produce increased strain on muscles and are usually uncomfortable for the client.***
2. Wrong choice. The longest, strongest muscles are less likely to become injured than the small

muscles, so this action uses good body mechanics. The question asks you to identify something the nurse would AVOID doing. Make another selection.

3. *Wrong choice. Body weight adds force to muscle action when pushing any object. This is a correct action, using good body mechanics. The question asks you to identify something the nurse would AVOID doing. Make another selection.*
4. *Wrong choice. When objects are close to the body, the line of gravity is within the body's base of support, which improves balance and reduces strain on the arm muscles. Carrying objects close to the body (without touching your clothing) uses good body mechanics. The question asks you to identify something the nurse would AVOID doing. Make another selection.*

30. An elderly client is admitted to the hospital with pneumonia. His daughter, who takes care of him at home, says to the nurse, "I'm so glad he is here. You can take much better care of him than I can." The best nursing response to the daughter is:

1. "We do have the equipment and people to take care of sick clients."
2. "It is not easy to care for the elderly. How do you manage?"
3. "Sir, your daughter takes good care of you at home, doesn't she?"
4. "Are you feeling guilty because your father has pneumonia?"

1. *Incorrect. This response does not focus on the appropriate person, because the daughter has expressed her feelings to the nurse and is therefore the client in this case scenario. This response also focuses on inappropriate issues concerning other people and hospital equipment. To be therapeutic, the nurse's response should focus on the daughter's feelings and concerns.*
2. ***Very good! This response uses the communication tool of showing empathy, and asks for clarification of the statement made to the nurse.***

> ***TEST-TAKING TIP:*** *Be sure to correctly identify the client in communication questions! The daughter is the client in this question, and the nurse's response should address her concerns. Note that Options 1 & 3 focus on inappropriate issues, and Option 4 implies to the client that she may be to blame for her father's pneumonia.*

3. *Incorrect. This response is not directed towards the appropriate person! The father is the person with the medical problem, but his daughter, who has expressed her feelings to the nurse, is the client in this test question. The nurse's response should be addressed to the daughter.*
4. *Incorrect. This response may appear to place blame on the daughter for her father's pneumonia. This type of response can put the client on the defensive, which is not therapeutic. Remember, the daughter is the client in this question.*

31. A client has pregnancy induced hypertension. In planning care for this client prior to delivery, which is most the most essential nursing order?

1. Assess fluid balance hourly and maintain optimum placental perfusion.
2. Monitor urine output and assure a brief rest period every shift.
3. Check the blood pressure before and after each time the client is out of bed.
4. Observe for amount of edema and provide for diversionary activities.

1. ***Excellent! Fluid balance has a relationship to blood pressure and should be assessed frequently. Assessment of fluid balance should include recording of intake and output, measurement of blood pressure, and observation of amount of edema. To maintain optimum placental perfusion, the nurse should assist the client to turn from side to side, but remain in a lateral position. This is the most essential nursing order for this client's plan of care. This question uses the planning phase of the nursing process.***
2. *Incorrect. Monitoring urine output is an important assessment because oliguria could indicate renal damage in a client with pregnancy induced hypertension, but output should be monitored more frequently than once a shift! Also, the client should be on bed rest to decrease the need for oxygen by the cells, which will decrease cardiac workload. A brief rest period every shift is not adequate. Try again.*
3. *Incorrect. It is true that the blood pressure should be monitored frequently; if the blood pressure is too high, drugs may be used to control it. The client should not be getting out of bed for activities, however, bed rest is necessary to decrease the need for oxygen by the cells, which will decrease cardiac workload. Try again.*
4. *Wrong choice. The nurse should observe for the amount of edema and should provide diversionary activities for the client. This is not, however, the most essential nursing order for this client. Try again.*

32. A 22-year-old client sustained a T-4 spinal cord injury. While doing morning assessments four weeks post-injury, the nurse discovers his BP is 280/140 and he is complaining of nasal stuffiness and a severe, pounding headache. The first nursing action is to:

1. Sit the client upright.
2. Call the physician.

3. Check the client's bladder for distension.
4. Administer the prescribed antihypertensive.

1. ***Correct choice! Since autonomic hyperreflexia is a medical emergency, the first action is to lower the BP. By sitting the client upright, compensatory orthostatic hypotension is used to lower the BP.***

2. Incorrect. This is not the first nursing action. Calling the physician is important after nursing measures have been initiated to lower the BP. What should the nurse do first?

3. Incorrect. This should be done to assess the cause of hyperreflexia, but the first goal is to lower the BP and, ultimately, to prevent stroke. What should the nurse do first?

4. Incorrect, because causing orthostatic hypotension will provide the same results initially. Antihypertensives are used only if nonpharmacologic methods are unsuccessful. What should the nurse do first?

33. A client is in the hospital with renal failure. She is on fluid restriction. Which nursing measure is inappropriate?

1. Provide a variety of fluids in small containers.
2. Inform the client and family about the restriction.
3. Allow the client to help keep a record of oral intake.
4. Provide fluids only during meal times.

1. Wrong choice. This is an appropriate nursing measure that allows for choices and variety. Look for something the nurse should NOT do.

2. Wrong choice. Informing the client and the family of the restriction is an appropriate nursing action that will make compliance with the restriction more likely. The stem of the question is asking for something the nurse should NOT do.

3. Wrong choice. This is an appropriate nursing action that promotes participation of the client in her own care. The stem of the question is asking for something the nurse should NOT do.

4. Good work, you have identified the inappropriate action. Since the client may become thirsty at times other than meal times, this nursing measure can lead to noncompliance on the part of the client and family.

34. The physician has ordered the client to be discharged on a 2000 calorie diabetic diet. What is the most important nursing action in developing a teaching plan for this client's diet?

1. Obtain sample menus from the dietician to give to the client.
2. Ask the client to identify the types of foods that she usually eats and prefers.
3. Tell the client that she will have to change all of her previous eating habits.
4. Advise the client to buy only dietetic foods.

1. Sample menus may be helpful in providing the client with ideas for new foods or exchanges. This is not the most important nursing action in developing a diet teaching plan for this client. Make another choice.

2. Excellent! Asking the client what types of foods she prefers provides an opportunity for the nurse to include these foods in the client's diet, which will promote compliance.

3. Incorrect. The client may have to change some of her eating habits, but not ALL of them! Telling the client what to do is inappropriate. This option also fails to give the client any useful information to use in complying.

> ***TEST-TAKING TIP:*** *Note that the absolute word "all" in this option is a clue that this is probably an incorrect option.*

4. Incorrect. Fresh fruits and vegetables and many other unprepared foods are permitted in a diabetic diet, and the diabetic may also use some prepared foods that are not labeled "dietetic." This option is also incorrect because there are not enough dietetic foods available to meet all of the client's dietary requirements. Try again.

35. An eight-year-old client was admitted to the hospital with a diagnosis of acute rheumatic fever. Immediately after admission, which nursing assessment is most important?

1. Auscultation of the rate and characteristics of heart sounds.
2. Determining the location and severity of joint pain.
3. Identifying the degree of anxiety related to the diagnosis.
4. Determining the family's emotional and financial needs.

1. Correct. This is the priority assessment because tachycardia and cardiac murmur indicate cardiac involvement, which may lead to serious and life-threatening complications.

2. Wrong choice. Pain in one or more joints is characteristic of rheumatic fever and would be of concern to the nurse. Since joint pain is not life-threatening and since there are usually no permanent sequelae, this is not the priority assessment.

3. Wrong choice. Anxiety related to the diagnosis of rheumatic fever and the symptoms and treatment of rheumatic fever is expected and would be of concern to the nurse. This anxiety is not life-threatening and would not receive top priority during the initial assessment.

4. *Wrong choice. The family's emotional needs at this time are of concern to the nurse. The length and cost of the treatment needed for rheumatic fever may place a burden on the family's emotional and financial resources, however, this would not be the top priority during the initial assessment of the child.*

36. A client recently diagnosed with multiple sclerosis questions the nurse concerning the usual course of the disease. What would be the most appropriate response by the nurse?

1. "Each client is different. We cannot tell what will happen."
2. "I can see that you are worried, but it's too soon to predict what will happen."
3. "Usually, acute episodes are followed by remissions, which may last a long time."
4. "It's too early to think about the future; let's focus on the present and go day-by-day."

1. *Wrong response. This provides no information to the client and blocks further communication. Try again.*
2. *Incorrect. The nurse acknowledges the client's feelings, but then blocks communication by failing to providing any information to help address her fears. Choose another option.*
3. ***Good choice! The nurse provides factual information while giving the client some realistic hope.***
4. *Incorrect. Remember that giving advice is a block to communication and will stop the client from feeling free to express concerns and fears. Choose again.*

37. While transferring a client with left-leg weakness from the bed to a wheelchair, the priority nursing action is to:

1. Have the seat of the wheelchair at a right angle to the bed.
2. Lock the wheels on the bed and the wheelchair.
3. Allow the client to do as much as possible to increase his sense of independence.
4. Have the client lock his hands around the nurse's neck to provide the client with a sense of security.

1. *Incorrect. This position would require the client to pivot 180 degrees to get into the seat of the wheelchair. The seat of the wheelchair should be parallel with and close to the bed for ease of access for the client. Try again.*
2. ***Correct! Locking the wheels of both bed and wheelchair provides for the client's safety by not allowing the equipment to move away from the client, thereby risking an injury from a fall.***

> ***TEST-TAKING TIP:*** Maslow's Hierarchy of Needs indicates that when there is no immediate physiological need, safety needs receive priority.

3. *Incorrect. Although encouraging independence is important, the client's safety is the most important consideration. A client with a weakened lower extremity is at risk for falling. Try again.*
4. *This action is unsafe! The client can place his hands on the shoulders of the nurse, but not around her neck. If the client slips, all of client's weight will be placed on the cervical vertebrae of the nurse, which could cause a spinal cord injury. Try again.*

38. The nurse enters the room and finds a mother crying. Her son has been diagnosed with leukemia and is currently receiving chemotherapy. The mother says, "I just can't believe he's going to lose all his beautiful blonde hair!" Which response by the nurse is most justifiable?

1. "Sometimes the hair only thins."
2. "You're feeling a lot of loss right now."
3. "Remember, hair loss means the chemotherapy is working!"
4. "Kids love to wear the special baseball caps we have."

1. *Incorrect. While this statement may be true, this is not therapeutic for the mother at this time, as it minimizes her concerns and feelings and may discourage further communication.*
2. ***Good work! This empathetic statement validates the mother's feelings and encourages further communication.***
3. *Incorrect. Hair loss occurs because chemotherapy destroys rapidly growing cells, which include hair, linings of the GI tract, and cancer cells. It is not an indication of the effectiveness of the chemotherapy. This response contains inaccurate information and fails to address the client's feelings. This response is not therapeutic for the mother.*
4. *Wrong! This response is not therapeutic because it does not address the mother's feelings and concerns. It is also not helpful to generalize for all children.*

39. A client says to the nurse, "I am so frustrated with having five kids. My husband won't do anything to help me keep from getting pregnant." Which is the best nursing action initially?

1. Refer the client and spouse to family planning services.
2. Find out if the client could use a contraceptive that would not involve her husband.
3. Assess what the client means by "being frustrated."

4. Ask the client if her husband is interested in birth control.

1. Incorrect. Referring both of them to family planning services might be an option, but this option is not the best choice for the first action the nurse should take. What should the nurse do first?
2. Good job! Before planning anything, the nurse needs to get more information. Assessment is the first step of the nursing process.
3. Wrong. Although this response might appear to be a good choice because it uses clarification, the client has already stated that her frustration is due to the number of children. The nurse does not need to assess any more about the client's feelings of frustration. Try again.
4. This is incorrect because the client has already stated that her husband is not interested in birth control measures that directly involve him.

40. An adult client is diagnosed with pneumonia and is being treated with penicillin G sodium 3 million units IV every four hours. When completing the drug history, it is especially important for the nurse to assess the client for allergies to which medications?

1. Antituberculars.
2. Calcium channel blockers.
3. Aminoglycosides.
4. Cephalosporins.

1. Incorrect. There is no known cross-sensitivity between penicillin and antitubercular medications. Try again.
2. Wrong choice. There is no evidence of cross-sensitivity between penicillin and calcium channel blockers. Select another response.
3. Incorrect choice. There is no known cross-sensitivity between penicillin and aminoglycosides, which is another group of antibiotics.
4. Good choice! The issue in this question is cross-sensitivity. Many clients who are allergic to penicillins are also allergic to cephalosporins, and vice versa. There is a significant risk of cross-sensitivity.

41. A client is gravida 5 para 4. During admission, the nurse assesses that contractions are occurring every two minutes and lasting approximately 45 seconds. The client says she has been in labor for approximately 10 hours. The priority assessment the nurse needs to make at this time is:

1. Time the client last ate.
2. Cervical dilatation.
3. Allergies to medications.
4. Vital signs.

1. Incorrect. The time the client last ate is not the priority assessment for this client. What is the issue in this question? Try again.
2. Great choice! Based upon your knowledge of the stages of labor, full dilatation usually takes approximately eight hours in a multi-gravida woman. Since this woman has already been in labor for 10 hours, your first priority is to assess cervical dilatation to best plan for a safe delivery.
3. Wrong choice, this is not your first priority. What is the issue in this question? Try again.
4. Incorrect. Although vital signs are important to assess in the mother and the fetus, if she delivers while you are taking them, the conditions for delivery may not be safe. What is the issue in this question? Try again.

42. A client is admitted to the hospital at 38 weeks of gestation with a large amount of bright red vaginal bleeding. A diagnosis of partial abruptio placenta is made. She is on the fetal monitor, and her vital signs are: FH 138 regular, BP 98/52, pulse 118, respirations 24, temperature 97.6° F. Assuming all of the following are ordered by the physician, the nurse should give first priority to which nursing action?

1. Abdominal-perineal prep.
2. Insert Foley catheter.
3. Sign informed consent for surgery.
4. Start an IV.

1. Incorrect. An abdominal prep can be delayed until just prior to the cesarean delivery, if it is done.
2. Wrong, try again. The Foley catheter can be inserted in the delivery room just prior to the delivery, if it is needed.
3. Incorrect. The consent form, if not signed immediately by the client, can be signed by a family member if the situation warrants. This is not the nurse's priority at this time.
4. Correct! Insertion of the IV line into this client is the first priority. She is at high risk for shock; if that occurs it will be very difficult to insert an IV catheter. Inserting the IV now is the first priority for safe care.

43. A 15-year-old client is being seen in the family planning clinic. She says to the nurse that she is nervous and has never had a pelvic examination before. The appropriate response by the nurse is:

1. "All you have to do is relax."
2. "It is only slightly uncomfortable."
3. "What part of the exam makes you nervous?"
4. "If you want birth control pills, then a pelvic exam is required."

1. This statement is trite, does not address the client's concerns, and blocks communication by using false reassurance. This response is not therapeutic.

2. *This response does not address the client's concerns and does not encourage further discussion. The response is not therapeutic.*
3. ***Very good! This response recognizes the client's feelings. It also uses the tool of clarification to encourage the client to tell the nurse more about her concerns. This response is therapeutic.***
4. *Incorrect. This statement is true in its literal sense, but the nurse does not know if the client wants birth control pills. Do not "read into" the question! More importantly, however, the client might interpret this statement as expressing disapproval by the nurse. It is non-therapeutic for the nurse to express approval or disapproval. This response also fails to address the feelings that the client has shared with the nurse. Try again.*

44. The first, most important nursing action when a nurse discovers a fire in a client's room is to:

1. Pull the fire alarm and notify the hospital operator.
2. Close fire doors and client room doors.
3. Remove the client from the room.
4. Place moist towels or blankets at the threshold of the door of the room with the fire.

1. *Wrong choice. Although pulling the fire alarm and alerting the hospital operator notifies the appropriate individuals who are needed to fight a fire, this is not the first nursing action. The immediate safety of the client in the room with the fire takes priority. Make another choice.*
2. *Wrong choice. Closing fire doors helps prevent the spread of a fire to other areas of the hospital, and closing the clients' room doors helps prevent smoke and fumes from entering their rooms. While this is an important intervention to help protect the other hospitalized clients, there is another action that should be implemented first. The immediate safety of the client in the room with the fire takes priority. Make another choice.*
3. ***Excellent! The client in the room with the fire is at highest risk for injury. The smoke from a fire can deprive a client of adequate oxygenation, and the fire poses a direct threat to the safety of this client. Moving this client to safety receives first priority.***
4. *Wrong choice. Although placing moist towels or blankets at the threshold of the door where the smoke is coming from helps prevent the smoke and fumes from entering other areas, this is an inappropriate action to take at this time. The client in the room with the fire is at risk for injury and oxygen deprivation. Try again.*

45. In assessing an adult client with diabetes mellitus, the nurse would identify which finding as unexpected with this diagnosis?

1. Possible increased body weight.
2. Increased urinary output.
3. Periods of polydypsia.
4. Altered heart rate and rhythm.

1. *Wrong choice. An adult diabetic may gain weight, so the word "possible" makes this a true statement. This question has a false response stem, so you are looking for a finding that is UNEXPECTED with this diagnosis. Try again!*
2. *Wrong choice. Increased urinary output is a manifestation of adult diabetes. This question has a false response stem, so you are looking for a finding that is UNEXPECTED with this diagnosis. Try again!*
3. *Wrong choice. Polydipsia is consistent with the diagnosis of adult diabetes. This question has a false response stem, so you are looking for a finding that is UNEXPECTED with this diagnosis. Try again!*
4. ***Very good! The question has a false response stem, so the answer is something that the nurse would NOT expect to find in an adult diabetic. Altered heart rate and rhythm are NOT characteristic of diabetes. The other three options are distractors: they list signs and symptoms consistent with the diagnosis of adult diabetes mellitus.***

46. A client is to be up in a chair three times a day. He is paralyzed from the waist down. What is the best nursing approach when transferring the client from a bed into a wheelchair?

1. Place the wheelchair close to the foot of the bed.
2. Utilize the principles of body mechanics while providing a safe transfer for the client.
3. Slide the client to the edge of the bed, keeping the nurse's back straight and using a rocking motion to pull the client.
4. Place the nurse's arms under the client's axillae from the back of the client.

1. *Incorrect. The wheelchair should be placed as close to the position of the client's buttocks as possible for a safe and easy transfer. The wheelchair should not be placed at the foot of the bed!*
2. ***Very good! The nurse is in control of the nurse's own body and the client's movement during the transfer. Providing for the safety of the client, and utilizing the principles of body mechanics to provide safety for the nurse, as well, is the best nursing approach.***

> ***TEST-TAKING TIP:*** *Options 3 and 4 describe specific actions that are correct in transferring a client, but Option 2 is the best option because it is a more comprehensive or global statement. When more than one option appears correct, look for a global response option.*

3. *Not the best choice. This is an appropriate nursing action that addresses the safety of the nurse and client. Positioning the client near the edge of the bed will reduce the energy required to move the client to the wheelchair, and the nurse's back will be protected by using leg and arm muscles to move the client to the edge of the bed. However, there is another option that better describes the "best nursing approach" in transferring this client. Try again.*
4. *Not the best choice. Supporting the upper portion of the client's body helps to place the weight of the client over the nurse's center of gravity. This is a correct action that helps provide for the nurse's and the client's safety. However, there is another option that better describes the "best nursing approach" in transferring this client. Try again.*

47. A client puts her call light on and tells the nurse that she has to urinate. The client has had a Foley catheter in place since her surgery two days ago. Which is the most appropriate nursing action initially?

1. Remind the client that she has a Foley catheter in place and does not need to go to the bathroom.
2. Replace the Foley catheter with a new catheter.
3. Explain to the client that the urge to void is a common occurrence for clients who have urinary catheters.
4. Check the catheter and tubing for kinks and note the urine output in the drainage bag.

1. *Incorrect. Although a Foley catheter is in place, it may not be patent, which can result in distention of the bladder and cause the client to feel the urge to void. This action by the nurse does not meet the client's needs. Try again.*
2. *Incorrect. A new catheter might be necessary to meet the client's needs, but the nurse must assess the situation further to determine the cause of the client's urge to void. Try again.*
3. *Incorrect. The urge to void usually occurs upon initial insertion of the Foley catheter, not two days afterwards. There are several possible reasons for the client having urgency, and the nurse must attempt to discover the cause in order to meet the client's needs. Try again.*
4. ***Yes! Checking the equipment is the best nursing action, since data will be obtained that will assist the nurse with problem solving.***

__TEST-TAKING TIP:__ This prioritizing question uses the nursing process. The nurse should always assess before planning or implementing a nursing intervention. The nurse does not know the reason for the client's need to void, which means that the implementation actions in Options 1, 2, and 3 cannot be the answer.

48. A 49-year-old client has been diagnosed with iron deficiency anemia. When teaching the client about her diet, the nurse should recommend an increased intake of:

1. Fresh fruits.
2. Milk and cheese.
3. Organ meats.
4. Whole grain breads.

1. *Wrong. Fruits are a good source of vitamins A and C; this client is deficient in iron. Try again.*
2. *Wrong. Dairy products are good sources of high quality complete protein, not iron. This option does not correctly address the issue in the question.*
3. ***Right choice! A diet rich in organ meats provides iron, which is what the client needs to improve her anemia.***
4. *Wrong. Whole grain breads are rich in carbohydrates and dietary fiber, not iron. This option does not correctly address the issue in the question.*

49. A client is to have a nasogastric tube inserted because of an obstruction in his bowel. The nurse explains the procedure to him and is about to begin the insertion, when the client says, "No way! You are not putting that hose down my throat. Get away from me." The best nursing response is:

1. "You have the right to refuse treatment. Why don't you talk to your doctor about it?"
2. "Something is upsetting you. Can you tell me what it is?"
3. "What exactly do you feel about this 'hose'?"
4. "It'll be easier for you to just get it over with. It only gets harder if you get worked up over it and you won't get better without this tube."

1. *Incorrect. This response puts the client's feelings on hold, referring them to another person at a later time. Although the client has the right to refuse treatment, the nurse should give him an opportunity to express his concerns. This response blocks communication. Try again.*
2. ***Very good. This response addresses the client's feelings. This option uses the communication tool of clarification, which helps the nurse assess the situation. It is more global than Option 3, which focuses only on the client's feelings about the nasogastric tube.***
3. *Incorrect. This option asks for a response from the client concerning the hose. The nurse does not need information concerning the hose. The nurse needs information concerning the client's feelings about the whole situation. Try again.*
4. *Incorrect. In this response, the nurse is blocking communication by giving advice. Try again.*

50. The nurse tells a client that the doctor has ordered an intravenous line to be started. The client ap-

pears to be upset but says nothing to the nurse. Which is the best nursing response?

1. "Do you have any questions about the procedure?"
2. "The doctor wants you to have antibiotics, and this method eliminates getting frequent injections."
3. "What is there about this procedure that concerns you?"
4. "It only hurts a little bit. It'll be over before you know it."

1. Not the best response. This response focuses too narrowly on the procedure. What is the issue in this communication question?

2. Wrong. This response focuses on an inappropriate person (the doctor) and raises an inappropriate issue (antibiotics by injection). This response does not promote therapeutic communication.

3. Very good! This response uses the communication tool of clarification and invites the client to express his concerns and feelings with the nurse.

4. This option is incorrect. An intravenous puncture hurts more than a little bit. This communication block is identified as false assurance. In this response the nurse is assuming that the client's silence stems from a concern about pain. Which option uses the communication tool of clarification and focuses on the client's feelings?

51. A client shows the nurse the result of his recent tuberculin skin test. The site is red and swollen. The nurse interprets this as:

1. The client has active tuberculosis.
2. The client has a history of tuberculosis.
3. The tubercle bacillus is in the active pulmonary stage of tuberculosis.
4. The client has had contact with the tubercle bacillus.

1. Wrong. A skin test that shows a marked change indicates only that the client was exposed to the tubercle bacillus. A positive chest x-ray and a positive sputum culture for the acid-fast bacillus would indicate active tuberculosis.

TEST-TAKING TIP: *Note that Options 1 and 3 are very similar. Two options that use the same idea must be distractors and can be eliminated.*

2. Wrong. A positive tuberculin skin test means only that they have been exposed to the tubercle bacillus. This does not indicate that they have had tuberculosis.

3. Wrong. A positive skin test does not indicate an active lesion. Further tests are necessary to diagnose active tuberculosis.

4. Correct! A marked reaction to the skin test only indicates exposure to the tubercle bacillus. This question requires an understanding of what a positive reaction to the tuberculin skin test indicates.

52. A client is in the hospital and has weakness on her left side because of a stroke. She becomes upset when eating because liquids drool out of her mouth on her weak side. What nursing intervention would be most appropriate?

1. Provide only pureed and solid foods to prevent drooling, in order to prevent the client from becoming upset.
2. Have a member of the family assist with the client's feedings.
3. Teach the client how to drink fluids on the unaffected side to prevent drooling.
4. Have the client use a syringe to squirt liquids into the back of her mouth.

1. Wrong. Eliminating liquids from the client's diet is inappropriate, since fluids are a basic physiological need.

2. Wrong. This option does not solve the problem of the drooling fluids and does not promote independence in this client.

3. Correct. This promotes independence and addresses the problem of drooling, which is the issue in this question. The client still has control over swallowing and tongue motion on the unaffected side.

4. Although this may help eliminate some drooling, it does not promote normalcy during eating, which can result in a decrease in self-esteem.

53. A 10-year-old boy is in sickle cell crisis. Which nursing action is contraindicated?

1. Administer oxygen via nasal cannula as prescribed.
2. Encourage the client to increase oral fluid intake.
3. Administer narcotics only for very severe pain.
4. Encourage as much exercise as possible during the crisis.

1. Incorrect choice; this action is appropriate. Hemoglobin S forms a sickled shape in the presence of low oxygen tension, and oxygen is administered to prevent the condition of low oxygen tension. You are looking for something the nurse should NOT do.

2. Wrong choice; this action is appropriate. High fluid intake prevents dehydration, which would encourage aggregation of the cells and microvascular occlusion. You are looking for something the nurse should NOT do.

3. Wrong choice; this action is appropriate. Relief of pain is an important goal during a sickle cell crisis, but physical measures, such as application of heat, should be used whenever they are effective. If physical measures are not effective, non-narcotic analgesics should be tried. Narcotics are administered only for severe pain that is not relieved by physical measures and non-narcotic analgesics. Clients with sickle cell anemia are likely to have pain over an extended period of time, and addiction may become a problem. You are looking for something the nurse should NOT do.

4. ***You are correct; the nurse should not encourage exercise! During a sickle cell crisis, exercise should be kept to a minimum. Clients are usually placed on bed rest to decrease the need for oxygen by the cells.***

> **TEST-TAKING TIP:** Note that the word "crisis" appears in the stem of the question and in this option. If you did not know the answer, this is a clue that this option might be correct. Be sure to always "go with what you know," however, that is always the best test-taking strategy!

54. A 21-year-old client has sustained a basal skull fracture. The nurse notices drainage from his right nostril. The priority nursing action is to:

1. Notify his physician.
2. Suction his nostril.
3. Test the drainage for glucose.
4. Ask the client to blow his nose.

1. *Incorrect. The nurse has not determined the source of the bleeding and does not have the information that the physician will require. What should the nurse do first?*
2. *Wrong! This is contraindicated if the drainage is cerebral spinal fluid. Try again.*
3. ***Good choice! Positive glucose on a reagent strip signifies that the drainage is cerebral spinal fluid. This must then be reported to the physician.***
4. *Incorrect. This is contraindicated because it may prolong closure of a dural tear and increase the risk of infection.*

55. If verapamil hydrochloride (Calan) is administered with propranolol (Inderal), the nurse should monitor the client closely for signs of:

1. Hypertension.
2. Increased peripheral resistance.
3. Bradycardia and heart failure.
4. Diarrhea.

1. *Incorrect. The client should be monitored for hypotension, not hypertension. Hypotension occurs as both drugs decrease myocardial contractions and lower peripheral resistance. Make another choice.*
2. *Incorrect. Increased peripheral resistance is the same concept as hypertension. The client should be monitored for hypotension, not hypertension. Hypotension occurs as both drugs decrease myocardial contractions and lower peripheral resistance.*

> **TEST-TAKING TIP:** When two options are similar, neither can be the correct answer.

3. ***Right! Bradycardia and heart failure can occur when these drugs are used together.***
4. *Wrong. Nausea and constipation are reported, but not diarrhea. Make another selection.*

56. In assessing a client after a bronchoscopy, the nurse would give immediate attention to:

1. Blood-tinged mucous.
2. Complaints of hoarseness when speaking.
3. Irritation and discomfort when swallowing.
4. Difficulty breathing.

1. *Incorrect. Blood-tinged mucous and sputum are normal after this procedure. The bronchoscope when inserted may cause trauma to the tissue of the larynx, trachea, or bronchi. This would not require immediate attention by the nurse.*
2. *Incorrect. The client may complain of hoarseness after the bronchoscopy because of the trauma to tissue of the larynx and the trachea. This complaint is normal after this procedure and would not require the nurse's immediate attention.*
3. *Incorrect. This is a normal symptom after a bronchoscopy. The swallowing reflex is usually blocked for about six hours after the procedure. Initially the client may have some discomfort and difficulty when the swallowing reflex is restored. This would not require the nurse's immediate attention.*
4. ***Yes! This is a priority assessment that needs immediate medical treatment. The difficulty in breathing may be caused by edema in the larynx or trachea and is a serious complication.***

57. The nurse is caring for a client who had abdominal surgery two days ago. Which assessment data requires immediate action by the nurse?

1. A urinary drainage bag with 100 ccs in a two-hour period.
2. A wound dressing with thick light green drainage.
3. A blood pressure reading of 98/66.
4. Shallow respirations, with a rate of 26.

1. *Wrong. The amount of urine in the drainage bag indicates adequate urinary output.*
2. ***Correct. Thick light green drainage is indicative of an infection and should be reported to the phy-***

sician immediately. The stem of the question requires analysis of the data by the nurse. This option also addresses a client safety issue, which requires an immediate response by the nurse.

3. *Wrong. Since baseline data is not provided in the question, the nurse cannot determine whether or not the blood pressure reading is normal for this client. Further assessment is needed.*
4. *Shallow respirations are not unusual for the client who has undergone abdominal surgery. Although the nurse needs to address this issue by having the client deep breathe and cough, it is not the priority action.*

58. A depressed client and her husband attend a client education class on the topic of depression and learn about the behaviors that could indicate a recurrence of depression. To evaluate the effectiveness of the teaching, the nurse asks the client to identify the indications of recurrence of depression. Which behavior or symptom if named by the client would indicate to the nurse that the client requires further instruction?

1. Psychomotor retardation.
2. Grandiosity.
3. Self-devaluation.
4. Insomnia.

1. *Wrong choice. Psychomotor retardation may be a sign of recurrence of depression, so this is not the answer. Look for the option that is NOT a sign of depression.*
2. ***Good work! Grandiosity is not associated with depression; it is associated with the manic phase of bipolar depression.***
3. *Wrong choice. Self-devaluation is associated with depression, so this is not the answer. Look for the option that is NOT a sign of depression.*
4. *Wrong choice. Insomnia or hypersomnia are two interrupted sleep patterns that are associated with depression. This is not the correct option because this negative response question is asking for an option that is NOT a sign of depression.*

59. An 18-month-old girl is admitted for a surgical repair of the cleft palate. She returns from the operating room supine, with an IV and a mist tent on room air. Which is the priority nursing action?

1. Medicate for pain.
2. Check the IV for signs of infiltration.
3. Turn the child on her side.
4. Review the postoperative orders.

1. *Wrong choice. The child may need medication for pain at some point, but this is not of immediate concern.*
2. *Wrong choice. The IV site should be checked frequently to assure patency and placement, but this is not of immediate concern.*
3. ***Yes! Airway is always an immediate priority. Turning the child on her side will protect the child from aspiration.***
4. *Wrong choice. The postoperative orders should be reviewed when the child is admitted to the acute care floor. This would not take precedence, however, over establishing a patent airway in a child at risk for aspiration.*

60. A male nurse received a doctor's order to catheterize one of his female clients. The client says, "I'm not going to allow a male nurse to catheterize me." The appropriate response by the nurse is:

1. "Your doctor is a male. Would you let him catheterize you?"
2. "I've done this many times with no problems."
3. "You can explain to your doctor why the catheter wasn't inserted."
4. "You appear to be upset. Let me find a female nurse to help with the procedure."

1. *This response is defensive, focuses on an inappropriate person (the doctor), focuses on an inappropriate issue (whether the client would allow the doctor to catheterize her), and devalues the client's feelings. This response places the client on the defensive and is not therapeutic.*
2. *This response is defensive, focuses on an inappropriate person (the nurse), focuses on an inappropriate issue (the nurse's competency), and does not address the client's feelings or concerns. This response is not therapeutic for the client.*
3. *This response is defensive, focuses on an inappropriate person (the doctor) and aggravates the problem. With this response, the nurse will fail to see that the required procedure is performed, which might endanger the client. This response is not professional.*
4. ***Good choice! This response shows empathy, responds to the client's concern and offers a possible solution to the problem. This is the best of the four options for this question. The other options are not client centered, are defensive, and do not respect client rights.***

61. A confused elderly client is found wandering around the ward wearing a bathrobe and cotton socks. He is bumping into walls as he walks. At this time, the nurse should:

1. Take the client's shoes to him and assist him in putting them on.
2. Accompany the client to his room and obtain a baseline assessment.
3. Ask the client to return to his room and rest until he feels better.

4. Tell the client to be careful of any wet spots on the floor.

1. *Wrong. In this option, the nurse fails to ensure the client's immediate safety. He is at risk of falling because of ambulating in stocking feet and bumping into walls. This option also does not address the issue of what is causing the client to bump into walls. Try again.*
2. ***Excellent! The nurse ensures the client's safety by accompanying him to his room. Assessment is also essential because the client's bumping into walls indicates impairment of the client's balance and level of consciousness, which may be a manifestation of an emerging complication. Good work!***
3. *Wrong. In this option, the nurse fails to ensure the client's immediate safety. Also, the nurse does not know that the client feels ill or will feel better later. The nurse needs more information.*
4. *The case scenario does not tell you anything about wet spots on the floor, and this option does not address the issue of the client's bumping into walls. The nurse must act to provide for the client's immediate safety, and the nurse needs more information to determine the cause of the client's behavior.*

62. A client, age 31, is brought to the Emergency Room after an automobile accident. She is conscious upon admission. A physical examination and x-rays reveal a transection of the spinal cord at T-4. The nurse should give the highest priority to which information?

1. The client has an allergy to iodine.
2. The client last voided seven hours ago.
3. The client smokes two packs of cigarettes a day.
4. The client is menstruating.

1. *Incorrect. Although this information may be important later, especially if any diagnostic tests using dye contrast media are ordered, it is not priority at this time. Look for an option that can be life-threatening to the client in this immediate situation.*
2. ***Excellent priority setting! A distended bladder is the most common cause of autonomic dysreflexia, an acute emergency that occurs as a result of exaggerated autonomic responses. It is characterized by severe, pounding headache with paroxysmal hypertension, profuse sweating, and bradycardia. Because this is an emergency situation, the objective is to remove the triggering stimulus as soon as possible.***
3. *Incorrect choice. This assessment is certainly important to validate the high risk for respiratory complications secondary to smoking; however, it's not the priority observation at this time. Look for an option that can be life-threatening to the client in this immediate situation.*
4. *No. The fact that the client is menstruating does not constitute an immediate emergency situation. Choose another option.*

63. A 25-year-old female client is taking ampicillin (Amcill) and birth control pills containing estrogen. What information should the nurse provide?

1. Take both medications with breakfast to avoid gastric upset.
2. When used together, serum potassium levels may rise.
3. The effectiveness of the birth control pills may be reduced while the client is taking ampicillin.
4. Urticaria is much more common when antibiotics are given with other drugs.

1. *Wrong! The effect of ampicillin is decreased slightly when taken with foods, so this would not be advisable. Try again.*
2. *Incorrect. Potassium levels are only monitored with IV penicillins that contain high amounts of potassium, such as Potassium Pen G. Try again.*
3. ***Good choice! The issue in this question is drug interaction. Estrogen metabolism is increased, or there is a reduction of enterohepatic circulation of estrogens, when ampicillin is taken by a woman using birth control pills. Another form of birth control should be used while a client is on ampicillin.***
4. *Incorrect. Urticaria occurs with sensitivities to all penicillins, regardless of whether another medication is being used. This option does not address the issue in the question, which is drug interaction. Make another choice.*

64. A client, 65 years old, is admitted to the hospital for surgery after finding a lump in his right testicle. He asks the nurse, "Do you think the doctor will find cancer?" Which is the best nursing response initially?

1. "Most lumps found in the testicles are benign."
2. "It must be difficult for you not to know what the doctor will find."
3. "I think that you should discuss this with your doctor."
4. "It might be, but the doctor won't know until the surgery is performed."

1. *This may be a true statement, but it does not allow the client to express his fears concerning cancer. This response blocks communication between the client and the nurse.*
2. ***Very good! This response promotes communication by allowing the client to express his feelings.***
3. *Referring the client's concern to the doctor puts the client's concern on hold and is not a therapeutic nursing response. The client's feelings and concerns need to be addressed by the nurse.*

4. *This response does not help the client to explore his feelings and is not a therapeutic nursing response.*

65. A client's psychiatrist orders lithium four times daily. When administering medications on the sixth day, the nurse notes that the client's laboratory report indicates a serum lithium level of 1.0 mEq/liter. Based on this lab report, the most appropriate nursing action at this time is to:

1. Withhold the next dose of lithium and notify the psychiatrist.
2. Ask that the laboratory test be repeated.
3. Assess the client for possible toxic effects.
4. Administer the next dose of lithium as ordered.

1. *Wrong. The lithium level is within the therapeutic range.*
2. *This is not necessary. The lithium level is within the therapeutic range.*
3. *Wrong choice. This is an appropriate nursing action, since the nurse should continuously assess the client's responses to medication. It is not, however, an action that the nurse would take "based on the lab report," because the report indicates that the lithium level is within the therapeutic range. The case scenario presents no information suggesting lithium toxicity. Do not "read into" the question — and be sure to read all the options before identifying the best one!*
4. ***Correct. The lithium level is within the therapeutic range. The next dose should be administered as ordered.***

> ***TEST-TAKING TIP:*** *If you could not select the correct option using your nursing knowledge alone, you could use the strategy of eliminating similar distractors in this question. Note that Options 1, 2, and 3 would be appropriate only if the level were outside the therapeutic range. Option 4 is the option that is different. This strategy is useful to know!*

66. A client is seen in the clinic in the 28th week of gestation. Her blood pressure is 160/100 and she has 2+ protein in her urine. She complains that all her shoes are too tight. Her doctor recommends hospitalization. The nurse who is admitting the client must select a bed for the new client. Each room on the unit is a semiprivate room. Which roommate should the nurse select for this client?

1. A 20-year-old primigravida who enjoys loud rock-and-roll music.
2. A 32-year-old multigravida who enjoys reading romance novels.
3. A 24-year-old C-section who watches soap operas and game shows on TV.
4. A 22-year-old primigravida who has many visitors during the afternoon and evening.

1. *Wrong. The client has symptoms of preeclampsia, including hypertension, proteinuria, and ankle edema. Because of the hypertension and danger of seizures, the best environment for her is one that will facilitate rest and relaxation. The roommate in this option will increase the noise in the environment. The same is true of the roommates in Options 3 and 4, and these similar distractors should be eliminated.*
2. ***You selected the right answer! The client has symptoms of preeclampsia, including hypertension, proteinuria, and ankle edema. Because of the hypertension, there is a danger of seizures. The best environment for her is one that will facilitate rest and relaxation. A roommate who likes quiet activities such as reading will be best.***

> ***TEST-TAKING TIP:*** *In each of the other three options, the roommate will increase the noise in the environment. These similar distractors should all be eliminated.*

3. *Wrong. The client has symptoms of preeclampsia, including hypertension, proteinuria, and ankle edema. Because of the hypertension and danger of seizures, the best environment for her is one that will facilitate rest and relaxation. The roommate in this option will increase the noise in the environment. The same is true of the roommates in Options 1 and 4, and these similar distractors should be eliminated.*
4. *The client has symptoms of preeclampsia, including hypertension, proteinuria, and ankle edema. Because of the hypertension and danger of seizures, the best environment for her is one that will facilitate rest and relaxation. The roommate in this option will increase the noise in the environment. The same is true of the roommates in Options 1 and 3, and these similar distractors should be eliminated.*

67. A client asks the nurse how relaxation techniques will help his gastric pain. "Can't I just take the Tagamet that my physician has prescribed?" In responding to his question, the nurse is guided by the knowledge that:

1. Gastric ulcer is a stress-related illness, and his stress levels and emotional issues are contributing to the exacerbation of his symptoms.
2. He is in denial, because he is refusing to acknowledge that stress is playing a role in the progress of his illness.
3. Gastric ulcer and other psychosomatic illnesses are caused by stress and can't be cured with only medical or surgical treatments.
4. The client is displaying the "typical ulcer personality" of a competitive, aggressive person who is defending against unresolved dependency needs.

1. ***Correct. The client's question indicates that he does not readily perceive the relationship between stress and the exacerbation of his ulcer. The nurse, guided by this knowledge, can formulate a response to help him better understand his illness.***
2. *Incorrect. The client's question does not necessarily indicate denial. Without additional assessment data not presented in this case scenario, the nurse cannot know whether the client is refusing to acknowledge the role of stress in his illness. Do not "read into" the question.*
3. *Incorrect. Stress alone does not cause a gastric ulcer. There are physiological factors that are more directly involved. Try again!*
4. *Incorrect. Current research indicates that a "typical ulcer personality" does not exist.*

68. A six-week-old infant with AIDS is being prepared for discharge. The child's primary caregiver is the grandmother. Which statement by the grandmother would alert the nurse to a need for further instruction?

1. "I know that handwashing is an important preventative measure."
2. "I'll use disposable diapers, discarding them in separate plastic bags."
3. "Blood spills should be washed up immediately with hot soapy water."
4. "Gloves should be worn by all persons changing the baby's diapers."

1. *Wrong choice. This response indicates the grandmother's understanding of transmission of the disease and the effectiveness of handwashing as an effective method of preventing infection to the client and to the family. This statement does not represent a hazard.*
2. *Wrong choice. This is an acceptable method of infection control. Any items that cannot be disposed of in the toilet should be kept in a closed plastic bag until trash disposal. This statement by the grandmother does not represent a knowledge deficit.*
3. ***Good work! This is an inadequate method of cleaning blood or potentially contaminated body substances. Bleach solution should be used and gloves worn whenever coming in contact with blood or other body substances.***
4. *Wrong choice. You do not need to follow up with the grandmother on this statement, because gloves should be worn by anyone when changing the diaper of a child who has tested HIV positive or has the AIDS virus. Blood and body fluids are a means of disease transmission.*

69. The most important nursing goal for a client who is admitted with an acute exacerbation of ulcerative colitis is:

1. To provide emotional support.
2. To prevent skin breakdown.
3. To maintain fluid and electrolyte balance.
4. To promote physical rest.

1. *Wrong choice. Emotional support is necessary, but physiological needs must be the priority in the acute stage.*
2. *Wrong choice. Preventing skin breakdown is important, but this is not the best statement of the "most important nursing goal" for this client. Read all the options before selecting the best one!*
3. ***Correct! Problems related to fluid and electrolyte balance can affect all systems. The primary goal would be to treat imbalances.***
4. *Incorrect. Rest promotes a decreased metabolic rate, but it is not sufficient to counteract problems resulting from fluid and electrolyte imbalances.*

70. The nurse observes a 72-year-old client trying to climb over the side rails of the bed. The nurse is placing a vest restraint on the client when the daughter arrives and says to the nurse, "My mother does not need to be tied down in bed. I've been caring for her for years, and she hasn't fallen out of bed yet." The best initial response by the nurse is:

1. "I just saw your mother trying to climb over the side rails. Since I am concerned about her falling and hurting herself, I think this is best for her safety."
2. "Tell me how you managed to care for her at home."
3. "Hospital policy requires restraint vests on clients who are at risk for falling. I just saw your mother trying to climb over the rails. You don't want her to get hurt, do you?"
4. "The elderly may become confused in an unfamiliar place and do things they wouldn't do at home. It is difficult to see her restrained. While you are with her, the restraints can be off. Let me know when you are ready to leave."

1. *Wrong. The client's safety is the issue in this question. Since the daughter and nurse are with her, she is not in immediate danger. It is important to note that the client in this test question is the daughter, and the nurse should address the daughter's statement. This response focuses on safety and restraints, and not on the client's (the daughter's) concerns about her mother being tied down.*
2. *Wrong. This response does not focus on the issue in the question, which is the client's feelings about restraints being placed on her mother. This option may be appropriate later in the conversation, but is not the best initial response.*
3. *Wrong. This response implies that the daughter is not interested in her mother's safety and makes*

her defensive. It focuses on hospital policy and not the daughter's concerns. The daughter is the client in this question, and the nurse's response must be therapeutic for the daughter.

4. ***Excellent! This option focuses on the daughter's concerns. It uses the therapeutic communication tool of empathy and provides information and rationales for the restraints. It also provides for safety and offers a compromise to the daughter that addresses her concerns and gives her some control.***

71. The nurse is caring for a client who is recovering from surgery. He has a urinary catheter in place that needs to be irrigated. The correct approach to prevent injury to the mucosa of the bladder is:

1. Gently compress the ball of the syringe to instill the irrigating solution.
2. Quickly instill the irrigating solution, using some pressure to loosen any clots or mucous.
3. After instilling the solution, apply gentle pressure to remove the irrigating solution from the bladder.
4. Place a sterile cap on the end of the drainage tubing to protect it from contamination.

1. ***Best choice! Gentle instillation creates a flow that helps to dilute and free sediment or debris within the lumen of the catheter.***
2. *No! Using force can injure tissue or cause the solution to leak from the connection. Any suction should be avoided because the mucosa of the bladder is easily injured. Removing the syringe from the catheter will break any suction created by vacuum. Note that Option 3 also involves the use of "pressure." Both of these options are wrong.*
3. *No! Using force can injure the mucosa of the bladder. Like Option 2, this distractor involves "pressure." This is a clue that both of these similar distractors are wrong.*
4. *Wrong choice. A sterile cap can help prevent a potential infection but does not protect the mucosa of the bladder from injury during irrigation. This option does not address the issue in the question.*

72. A 21-year-old client is admitted to the hospital because of extreme weight loss. It is noted on the admission assessment that the client believes that she is overweight at 88 pounds. What aspect of care should the nurse consider the first priority for this client's care?

1. Assessing the client's nutritional status.
2. Obtaining a psychiatric consult.
3. Planning a therapeutic diet for the client.
4. Talking to family members to find out more about the client's self-concept.

1. ***Excellent! The client's nutritional status should receive first priority, because nutrition is a basic physiological need. If the client's nutritional needs are not met, the situation may be life-threatening.***
2. *Wrong choice. Obtaining a psychiatric consult may be an appropriate intervention, but with only the information given in this case scenario, it would not take priority at this time. Make another selection.*
3. *Wrong choice. The client will need adequate nutrition and you are correct in identifying nutrition as a basic physiological need and a high priority. Planning nursing interventions should come after one of the other options in this question. Make another selection.*
4. *Wrong. Obtaining further information from the family may be appropriate, but it is not the priority action in this situation. Make another selection.*

73. A client is hospitalized for a closed reduction of a fractured femur and application of a cast. A vital nursing action in the care of this client is to:

1. Perform neurovascular checks of the extremities.
2. Use the palms of the hands when moving an extremity with a wet cast.
3. Provide an instrument for the client to scratch the itching areas of skin under the cast.
4. Petal the edges of the cast to provide smooth edges.

1. ***Excellent! This is an important aspect of care for the client with a fracture. Circulation can become compromised and cause nerve and tissue damage. This action is more "vital" than the other three options.***
2. *Wrong choice. Using fingertips on a wet cast can cause indentations in the cast, resulting in pressure areas inside the cast. Although using the palms is an appropriate nursing action, it is not the most important or "vital" action. Read all the options, and make another choice.*
3. *Wrong! This is not an appropriate nursing action! Scratching under the cast can cause injury to the skin and potential infection. Try again.*
4. *Wrong choice. Although petaling the edges of the cast should be done to prevent injury to the skin caused by uneven edges of the cast, this is not the most important or "vital" nursing action.*

> *__TEST-TAKING TIP:__ This answer is similar to another choice in that it concerns care of the cast. When you cannot select the best option, a good strategy is to eliminate similar distractors.*

74. After detoxification, a client begins the rehabilitation phase of treatment. He tells the nurse that he

cannot imagine living his life without alcohol. The nurse's best response is based on what knowledge?

1. He will be more successful if he focuses on goals for short periods of time such as "today" or "this week".
2. He is likely to drink again when under stress.
3. He will not be successful if he is not strongly motivated.
4. He may require treatment with Antabuse to maintain sobriety.

1. ***Correct. Clients are less overwhelmed by the thought of sobriety when they set short-term goals that focus on "today" or "this week." Dealing with shorter periods of time is more manageable. The AA maxim, "One day at a time" is a reflection of this principle.***
2. *This might be true, but it is not the basis for a therapeutic response for this client.*
3. *This is not the best option. Motivation, without the development of needed skills, will not help the client to maintain sobriety.*
4. *Incorrect. Antabuse is used for individuals who lack the ability to abstain from alcohol without fear of adverse consequences. There is no data to indicate that this client requires Antabuse, since he is just beginning his rehabilitation program. Do not "read into" the question!*

75. While performing a vaginal exam on an obstetrical client, the nurse notes a glistening white cord in the vagina. The first nursing action is to:

1. Return to the nurses' station to place an emergency call to the physician.
2. Start oxygen at six to 10 liters, and assess the client's vital signs.
3. Cover the cord with a sterile moist saline dressing.
4. Apply manual pressure on the presenting part and have the mother get into a knee-chest position.

1. *Wrong choice. The physician needs to be called, but this is not the first priority — the health of the fetus is! What should the nurse do FIRST?*
2. *Wrong choice. This would not be helpful! All the oxygen in the world is not going to help this fetus if it cannot get it through the umbilical cord. The mother's vital signs are not a concern with a prolapsed cord; the fetal heart rate is of grave concern.*
3. *Not the best choice! Covering the cord with a moist sterile dressing will keep the cord moist and sterile, but it will not oxygenate the fetus.*
4. ***Yes! It is essential to get any pressure off the umbilical cord to allow oxygen to get to this fetus. Manual pressure on the presenting part and a knee-chest position are two ways to relieve umbilical cord compression.***

76. A client is in the hospital and has just found out that her mother died of a heart attack. She is crying and has her face buried in the pillow. The most therapeutic nursing response is to:

1. Return in fifteen minutes to see how the client is doing.
2. Sit with the client for a little while.
3. Tell the client that she will feel better in the morning.
4. Share with the client that the nurse's mother died within the last year and that the nurse knows just how she feels.

1. *Incorrect. This response does not promote therapeutic communication for the "here and now" of this question. The action indicates to the client that the nurse is not willing to offer self by staying with her during this stressful time. If the client wanted to communicate, there wouldn't be anyone to listen.*
2. ***Very good! The nurse lets the client know that she is important by providing time for her. Being silent is a communication tool that is appropriate during times of grieving. This response also addresses the "here and now" in this question.***
3. *Incorrect. This response devalues the client's feelings and puts them on hold. This response does not encourage therapeutic communication. It also offers false assurance, since she may not feel better in the morning.*
4. *Incorrect. This response focuses on an inappropriate person, the nurse, instead of the client's feelings. When the nurse expresses complete understanding of how the client feels, it inhibits communication, since this implies that there is no need for the client to express her own feelings. There is also an assumption by the nurse that grieving is the same for everyone.*

77. A client with asthma is receiving an oxygen concentration of 35%. The nurse knows that achievement of the therapeutic goal of this treatment is best demonstrated by:

1. Absence of adventitious breath sounds.
2. PaO2 92.
3. Heart rate increase of 25 beats/min.
4. Bicarbonate level of 25 mEq/liter.

1. *No, this is not the best indicator of oxygen therapy treatment. The absence of adventitious breath sounds means that crackles and wheezing are not audible, but does not tell you if there is adequate gas exchange.*
2. ***Correct. The goal of oxygen therapy is achievement of a PaO2 above 80 and no signs or symptoms of oxygen toxicity. This is a good example of a test question that uses the evaluation phase of the nursing process.***

3. *No, the opposite should occur if the oxygen is effective. The myocardial workload should be decreased, allowing for a slowing of the heart rate. Try again.*
4. *Incorrect. The value given is a normal bicarbonate, but is not an indicator of the client's response to oxygen therapy. This value is used to detect acid-base deviations.*

78. The primary nurse learns that an obsessive-compulsive client has a full set of dentures because he eroded all his tooth enamel with his brushing rituals. He also brushes his tongue several times a day, and has developed several ulcerations on it. His nursing care plan should set which goal as the highest initial priority?

1. He will eliminate his brushing and mouth care rituals.
2. He will verbalize the underlying cause of his behavior.
3. He will seek out the nurse when he is feeling anxious.
4. He will reestablish healthy tissue in his mouth and tongue.

1. *This is not correct. This option is the goal of his treatment, but it is not the highest initial priority for his care.*
2. *Wrong choice. This may or may not be appropriate, as behavioral methods will most likely be used to treat the client's problems. This would not be the highest initial priority.*
3. *Wrong choice. This is an appropriate goal, but is not the highest initial priority for his care.*
4. ***Correct. Restoring physiological integrity is the highest initial priority for this client. This will be done while working on the long-term goal of decreasing the mouth care rituals.***

79. The nurse is informed during report that a postoperative client has not voided for eight hours. The initial nursing action is to:

1. Assist the client to the bathroom.
2. Place the client on a bed pan and pour warm water over her perineum.
3. Palpate and percuss the client's bladder.
4. Catheterize the client.

1. *Assisting the client to the bathroom may be helpful if the client needs to urinate. This information needs to be obtained before action is taken. Make another choice.*
2. *Placing the client on a bed pan is not always conducive to urinating. If the client is allowed out of bed, sitting on the toilet while pouring warm water over the perineum can facilitate the client to void. However, this is not the priority action. The client should have the need and an urge to void before this intervention is implemented. Make another choice.*
3. ***Very good! Assessing the client's bladder provides information concerning the need to void. This is the priority action and the only option that provides for assessment of the client.***
4. *Catheterizing the client should only be done after it has been determined that the client has a full bladder and is unable to void. The nurse must assess first. Make another choice.*

80. A three-year-old is being admitted with nephrotic syndrome. The best roommate the nurse can select for this client is:

1. A 16-year-old recovering postoperatively from a ruptured appendix.
2. An eight-year-old with leukemia.
3. Another toddler with rheumatic fever.
4. No roommate, isolation is required.

1. *Wrong. The child with nephrotic syndrome is at risk for infection.*
2. ***Right. This child is not infectious, which is what the nurse is looking for as a roommate for a child with nephrotic syndrome. The roommates may have nothing in common, but the potential for infection is a high priority nursing diagnosis for this admission.***
3. *Wrong. The child with rheumatic fever may still be infectious from the original causative organism, and the child with nephrotic syndrome is at risk for infection.*
4. *No, it is not necessary to place this child on isolation. Try again.*

81. A client is to receive antibiotics. The priority nursing action when preparing to administer this medication is to:

1. Determine if the client has any allergies.
2. Determine the route of administration.
3. Check the client's name band.
4. Check the dosage against the physician's order.

1. ***Excellent choice! An allergy to an antibiotic can cause serious side effects. This is the priority nursing action, since the safety of the client is the issue.***

> ***TEST-TAKING TIP:*** *This option assesses before implementing. Use the nursing process when answering test questions!*

2. *Wrong; this is not a nursing action! The physician determines the route of administration, while the nurse implements the order. If there is a question about the route, the nurse needs to clarify the order. Which of the options represents the priority nursing action?*

3. *Wrong choice. The client's name band should be checked before administering any medication. The priority nursing action in preparing to administer the medication, however, is to note any allergies, especially when the medication is an antibiotic.*
4. *Wrong choice. Determining that the dose is correct is a nursing standard for medication preparation. If the client is allergic to the medication, however, the nurse need not prepare it. Notifying the physician of this fact is the next step and the priority nursing action.*

82. Before administering lithium, the nurse checks the client's latest lab report for her serum lithium level. She notes a level of 1.2 mEq/L. What is the best action for the nurse to take next?

1. Administer the next prescribed dose of lithium.
2. Suggest the blood test be repeated.
3. Withhold the next dose of lithium and notify the psychiatrist of the lab results.
4. Ask the client how he is feeling, to identify any untoward effects.

1. *Although the lithium level is still within the therapeutic range, it is at the very top of the range. This action is a possibility, but it could be unsafe. Read the other options to see if there is a better choice.*
2. *This action could be appropriate, but it is not the best action for the nurse to take next. Read the other options.*
3. *This is not correct. The lithium level is still within the normal range, so withholding the lithium is not an appropriate nursing action.*
4. ***Correct! A lithium level of 1.2 mEq/L is at the top of the therapeutic range. Before the nurse can safely give the next dose, she must assess the client for any signs of lithium toxicity. If the client has none, she can give the medication as prescribed.***

83. A client is admitted to the psychiatric unit with a diagnosis of acute depression. After being hospitalized for a few weeks, the client says to the nurse, "I'm a terrible person, and I should be dead." Which response by the nurse is appropriate initially?

1. "That is why you are here. We are trying to help you with your bad feelings."
2. "Feeling that way must be awful. What makes you feel so terrible?"
3. "Feeling like a terrible person is part of your illness. As you get better, those feelings will lessen."
4. "You are not terrible. You are not a bad person."

1. *Incorrect. This response appears to support the client's feelings that she is a terrible person. The second part of the response also blocks therapeutic communication by focusing on inappropriate persons: the nurse and others who "are trying to help" the client. This response is not therapeutic.*
2. ***Good choice! This response shows empathy, and then seeks clarification of the client's feelings. These two communication tools combine to make a therapeutic response that allows the client to talk about her feelings.***
3. *Wrong! This response gives information about the illness. At this time, the client's feelings must be addressed before information is given. When a client is distressed and upset, giving an explanation is inappropriate.*
4. *This response is not therapeutic for the client. The nurse's opinion is not important! This response blocks therapeutic communication by putting the nurse in the role of an authority figure, using false reassurance, and devaluing the client's feelings. The nurse's response should encourage the client to explore her feelings with the nurse.*

84. The nurse in a long-term care facility finds an elderly client on the floor. After having the client examined by the physician, the most important nursing action is to:

1. Call the family to stay with the client.
2. Provide for the safety and protection of the client.
3. Apply wrist and leg restraints to prevent the client from falling out of bed.
4. Obtain an order for medication to sedate the client.

1. *Having a member of the family stay with the client may be a possibility if it can be arranged. This provides for the client's safety and allows some mobility for the client while in bed. However, this is not the best option. Try again.*
2. ***Excellent! This global response option in effect includes providing all appropriate interventions that address the safety needs of the client. Maslow's Hierarchy of Needs indicates that the client's safety receives highest priority when no basic physiologic need is identified.***
3. *Application of restraints may be appropriate to ensure the safety of the client. A vest restraint would be more appropriate, however, since it provides mobility for the client and is less likely to cause agitation of the client. This is not the correct answer because wrist and leg restraints are not the first nursing action. Select another option.*
4. *Sedating a client often makes the client more confused and more likely to behave inappropriately. Other measures should take priority over sedation. Make another choice.*

85. A 25-year-old man was admitted one week ago with a diagnosis of schizophrenia, paranoid type. Since his admission, he has had several verbal outbursts of anger but has not been violent. A staff member tells the nurse that the client is pacing up and down the hall very rapidly and muttering to himself in an angry manner. The best initial nursing action is to:

1. Prepare an intramuscular injection of haloperidol (Haldol) to give him p.r.n.
2. Observe the client's behavior and approach him in a non-threatening manner.
3. Gather several staff members and approach the client together.
4. Contact the client's psychiatrist and request an order to place him in seclusion.

1. *Wrong! The client may need a p.r.n. dose of an antipsychotic if he is not able to control his behavior, however, this is not the best initial nursing action. Select a better option.*
2. ***Correct. The nurse must first assess the client's condition before deciding on an appropriate intervention. The best initial action is to approach him calmly, in a non-threatening manner, to ask him to verbalize what is bothering him.***
3. *Although it is important to have sufficient staff available to handle a potentially unsafe situation, there is a better option that more specifically addresses the approach the nurse should take initially.*
4. *This is not correct. The case scenario does not indicate that this intervention is needed.*

86. Betamethasone (Celestone) is administered to a client at 30 weeks gestation to reduce the risk of RDS in the neonate. The infant is born after two injections are given. In planning nursing care for the infant, which finding should be anticipated as a result of the administration of betamethasone to the mother?

1. Rapid pulse rate.
2. Sternal retractions.
3. Hypoglycemia.
4. Hypothermia.

1. *Incorrect. Betamethasone administration given to the antepartum client does not have an effect on neonatal vital signs. If this neonate has a rapid apical pulse, it is related to another cause, most likely his/her prematurity.*
2. *Incorrect. While it is quite likely that this premature neonate will have some RDS manifested by sternal retractions, it is most likely a result of immature lung development, and not related to the administration of betamethasone.*
3. ***Excellent! Betamethasone causes hyperglycemia in the mother, which predisposes the neonate to hypoglycemia in the first hours after delivery. This question concerns the planning phase of the nursing process and requires a knowledge of pharmacokinetics.***
4. *Incorrect. Betamethasone does not have any effect on the neonate's ability to maintain body temperature. If hypothermia is present, it is related to another cause, probably immature temperature regulation.*

87. In preparing to begin an aminophylline infusion, which nursing approach would be best?

1. Prepare a solution containing enough drug to last 24 hours.
2. Obtain an infusion pump to regulate the flow of the drug.
3. Insert a large IV catheter to assure adequate dilution.
4. Initiate measurement of intake and output to detect fluid retention.

1. *Wrong! Since aminophylline can be very toxic if infused too quickly, the total daily dose should be divided into several IV containers. If the infusion rate increases, a limited amount of drug will be infused.*
2. ***Yes! Since aminophylline can be very toxic if infused too quickly, a pump should be used to regulate the flow of this drug.***

> ***TEST-TAKING TIP:*** *Note that the word "infusion" appears in the stem of the question and in this correct option. When you don't know the answer and other strategies do not apply (looking for a global response, and eliminating similar distractors), a repeated word or phrase can be a clue that this is the correct answer.*

3. *Wrong! The size of the IV catheter is not relevant to dilution of the drug. The drug is diluted in the IV solution, not in the vein.*
4. *Wrong. I&O should be monitored, but the nurse will be looking for dehydration rather than fluid retention, since aminophylline acts as a diuretic.*

88. A client is being given an aminoglycoside for his bacterial infection. The nurse can aid in minimizing the risk of aminoglycoside toxicity by:

1. Weighing the client daily.
2. Encouraging the client to drink at least 2000 ml of fluids daily.
3. Monitoring blood pressure prior to drug administration.
4. Instructing the client to take the medicine with food.

1. *Incorrect. Although daily weights are an assessment tool useful in monitoring fluid volume deficit or excess, this action doesn't directly address*

the major concern with aminoglycosides. Try another response.

2. ***Good choice! Aminoglycosides accumulate in the kidneys, which is their site of excretion. Hydration serves to reduce the extent to which these drugs will be concentrated in the renal tubules, which can lead to renal toxicity. Remember that this intervention may be contraindicated in clients with a history of decreased renal function.***
3. *Incorrect. Hypertension is not a symptom of aminoglycoside toxicity. Make another selection.*
4. *Wrong. Aminoglycosides are poorly absorbed from an intact intestinal tract, but are rapidly absorbed intramuscularly. The only oral uses of aminoglycosides are for surgical prophylaxis ("bowel sterilization") or treatment of intestinal infections. Choose again.*

89. A client is hospitalized for gastrointestinal bleeding and is being treated with temazepam (Restoril). After the client's physician examined him, the nurse noted the physician wrote an order for the client to begin taking amitriptyline (Elavil). Which action by the nurse would be best initially?

1. Revise his medication schedule so that the Elavil is administered during the day and the Restoril at bedtime.
2. Monitor the client's vital signs closely.
3. Question the physician about administering both Elavil and Restoril to the client.
4. Assess the client for signs and symptoms of depression.

1. *Incorrect. Elavil is a tricyclic antidepressant that is very sedating. It is often chosen for depressed clients who also have difficulty sleeping. Restoril, a benzodiazepine, potentiates the effect of Elavil. The issue in this question is drug interaction. Try again.*
2. *This is not the best option. Although the client's vital signs should be monitored when he is placed on Elavil because it may cause orthostatic hypotension, this is not the initial nursing action in this case scenario. The issue in this question concerns drug interaction. Try again.*
3. ***Correct. Benzodiazepines, such as Restoril, potentiate the effects of other central nervous system depressants, such as the tricyclic Elavil. The nurse should contact the physician to question the safety of administering these two medications to the client.***
4. *This is an appropriate nursing action, but it is not the best initial action. The issue in this question concerns a drug interaction. Review the choices again and select the better action.*

90. The nurse is caring for a client with a myocardial infarction who is taking chlorothiazide (Diuril) and digoxin (Lanoxin). Which diet would be most appropriate to include in this client's nursing care?

1. Diet low in sodium and saturated fats, high in potassium.
2. Diet low in unsaturated fats, sodium, and potassium.
3. Diet high in potassium, Vitamin C, and protein.
4. Diet low in sodium and saturated and unsaturated fats.

1. ***Good choice! Sodium would be restricted to decrease the circulating blood volume and reduce the cardiac workload. Saturated fats would be decreased to prevent further atherosclerotic heart disease. Potassium should be increased in the diet because Diuril causes the excretion of potassium in the urine. It is vital to keep potassium within normal limits because a low potassium level may lead to arrhythmias in a client who is taking digoxin.***
2. *Incorrect! Both saturated and unsaturated fats are restricted in a weight reduction diet, however, the case scenario does not provide information that indicates this client needs to be placed on a weight reduction diet. Also, due to the drugs, loss of potassium can present a problem. Adequate potassium is needed to prevent cardiac arrhythmias.*
3. *Incorrect. A diet high in potassium is needed because of the loss of potassium due to digoxin and Diuril. There is no reason for increasing Vitamin C or protein.*
4. *Both saturated and unsaturated fats are restricted in a weight reduction diet, however, the case scenario does not provide information that indicates this client needs to be placed on a weight reduction diet. Also, due to the drugs, loss of potassium can present a problem. Adequate potassium is needed to prevent cardiac arrhythmias.*

91. The nurse is caring for a diabetic client who is currently taking cephalexin (Keflex). The nurse should advise the client that:

1. Clinitest or copper sulfate urine glucose tests give false positive results.
2. Blood sugar may drop without warning.
3. A source of sugar should always be carried with the client.
4. A medic alert bracelet should always be worn.

1. ***Correct. Cephalexin causes false positive results in urine glucose tests using cupric sulfate. Diabetic clients receiving cephalexin should use glucometers, or glucose enzymatic tests such as Clinistix.***
2. *Incorrect. This reaction is not caused by antibiotics. Make another selection.*

3. *Incorrect. This precaution is appropriate for all diabetics, regardless of whether they are on any medications. Look for an answer that relates to the effect of cephalexin on diabetics, which is the issue in the question.*
4. *All diabetics should wear a medic alert bracelet. This, however, does not address this client's need for advice regarding the effects of cephalexin.*

92. A client, age 82, is admitted to the psychiatric unit for a diagnostic work-up because she has become increasingly forgetful and disoriented at home. She has been taking lorazepam (Ativan) 0.5 mg p.r.n. to control her restlessness. In planning nursing care for this client, it would be unnecessary to include close observation for:

1. Orthostatic hypotension.
2. Increased anxiety.
3. Hyperexcitation.
4. Hallucinations.

1. ***Excellent choice! Orthostatic hypotension is a side effect of antipsychotics and tricyclic antidepressants. It is NOT a side effect of the benzodiazepines, like Ativan. This is the correct option because the stem is asking for an INCORRECT response.***
2. *Wrong choice. Increased anxiety is one of the symptoms of paradoxical excitement that can occur in elderly clients, so the nurse should closely observe for signs of increased anxiety. The stem in this question is asking for an INCORRECT response.*
3. *Wrong choice. Hyperexcitation is one of the symptoms of paradoxical excitement that can occur in elderly clients. This cannot be the correct option because the stem is asking for the symptom that does NOT occur with Ativan.*
4. *Wrong choice. Hallucinations are one of the symptoms of paradoxical excitement that can occur in elderly clients. It is not the correct option. Select the symptom that does NOT occur with Ativan.*

93. A client with chronic emphysema is taking theophylline (Theo-dur) at home. During the home care nurse's visit, which statement by the client would warrant immediate action?

1. "I just lie awake at night, worrying about the medical bills."
2. "I must have the flu. I was vomiting all night."
3. "I don't have my usual appetite. Nothing tastes good to me."
4. "I feel better if I have a big glass of milk with my pill."

1. *Insomnia is a common side effect of theophylline. While it is annoying and interferes with the client's rest, it is not life-threatening and does not call for immediate action.*
2. ***The client may indeed have the flu, but one of the early signs of theophylline toxicity is vomiting. Since there is no antidote for theophylline, and since toxicity can be fatal, the nurse should immediately explore other possible signs of toxicity and request a serum theophylline level.***
3. *A client receiving theophylline may have anorexia as a side effect of the drug. The client's nutritional status should be monitored. However, loss of appetite does not pose a life-threatening situation.*
4. *This statement indicates that the client understands how to minimize the gastric irritation caused by theophylline. There is no reason why milk cannot be taken with theophylline. Try again.*

94. A client, age 22, is admitted with a diagnosis of acute psychotic reaction, rule out schizophrenia. Because the client is very agitated, he is started on chlorpromazine (Thorazine) 100 mg t.i.d. After three days, he is much calmer and his nurse begins to teach him about his medication. Which statement by the nurse is most appropriate?

1. "This medication is a sedative to calm you down."
2. "This medication acts on the chemical regulators in your brain to help control your symptoms."
3. "This medication will cure your disorder."
4. "We do not know how this medication works, but we do know it will help you control your behavior."

1. *This is not an accurate statement. Antipsychotic medications like Thorazine may calm an agitated client, but they are not sedatives. They also control other symptoms of psychosis, such as delusions and other thought disturbances.*
2. ***Excellent! Antipsychotic medications are thought to act directly on the dopamine receptors in the brain to prevent the re-uptake of dopamine and thereby control psychotic symptoms.***
3. *This is not an accurate statement. Antipsychotics control symptoms but do not cure the psychotic disorder.*
4. *This is partially correct — but only partially! We do not know the exact mechanisms of action, but research has provided some information about how these drugs work. Antipsychotics block dopamine receptors in the brain, thereby controlling the target symptoms of psychosis. Read the options again to identify a better nursing response.*

95. A client scheduled for surgery the next day to create an ileal conduit is receiving neomycin sulfate (Mycifradin Sulfate). What is the nurse's best ex-

planation to the client for her receiving neomycin preoperatively?

1. To suppress of intestinal bacteria preoperatively, in order to decrease the risk of postoperative infection.
2. To decrease the number of pathogenic bacteria and decrease the number of loose stools.
3. To sterilize the bowel and prevent the risk of serious postoperative complications.
4. To prevent auditory impairment and nephrotoxicity during the postoperative period.

1. ***Yes, you are correct! Because bowel contents may spill during the bowel resection, suppression of intestinal bacteria is done preoperatively to reduce the risk of postoperative infection.***
2. *Wrong. While neomycin is sometimes used to treat diarrhea caused by Escherichia coli, there is no data to support this rationale for this client. Be careful not to "read into" the question! The issue is the preoperative use of neomycin in a client scheduled for an ileal conduit. Look for the option that correctly addresses that issue.*
3. *Wrong. Living tissue cannot be sterilized. Some organisms will remain.*
4. *Wrong. This answer does not make sense. Ototoxicity and nephrotoxicity are serious side effects of long-term neomycin treatment.*

96. A client, age 22, is admitted with pneumocystis carinii pneumonitis. The physician prescribes sulfamethoxazole trimethoprim (Bactrim), and a Foley catheter is inserted to monitor urinary output. Which nursing intervention would be most effective in reducing the risk of crystalluria secondary to sulfonamide therapy?

1. Encouraging fluid intake to 3000 cc/24 hours.
2. Irrigating the Foley catheter with normal saline every eight hours.
3. Monitoring specific gravity of urine every eight hours.
4. Providing foods/fluids likely to maintain an acidic pH of the urine.

1. ***Excellent choice! Maintenance of hydration ("natural irrigation") is the most effective intervention in preventing urinary stasis, which can lead to crystalluria. The client's output should be at least 1500 cc/day.***
2. *Incorrect choice. Irrigating a Foley catheter should never be a routine procedure because of the risk of infection created by interrupting a sterile system. There is a better and safer option. Select again.*
3. *Wrong choice. Monitoring the specific gravity of urine will give information regarding urine osmolality and the kidneys' ability to concentrate urine. It will not reduce the risk of crystalluria because it's only an assessment tool. Choose a more effective intervention.*
4. *Incorrect. The urine pH should be alkaline. Liquids and foods that produce acid urine should be avoided.*

97. A client is to receive IM methylergonovine (Methergine). In caring for the client, the nurse knows that the administration of IM Methergine is contraindicated in which situation?

1. Boggy fundus one hour after vaginal delivery.
2. Large amount of vaginal bleeding following abortion at 16 weeks.
3. Client with history of previous postpartum hemorrhage in recovery room.
4. Client who has not delivered placenta 20 minutes following birth of baby.

1. *No, this situation is an indication for the use of IM Methergine. A boggy fundus following delivery is indicative of uterine atony, which is treated by using an oxytocic drug such as Methergine. This question has a false response stem; so look for a CONTRAINDICATION.*
2. *No, this situation is an indication for the use of IM Methergine. A large amount of bleeding following an abortion usually indicates poor contractility of the uterus and is treated with an oxytocic drug. Remember, this question has a false response stem; so look for a CONTRAINDICATION.*
3. *No, this situation is an indication for the use of IM Methergine. Clients with a history of previous postpartum hemorrhage are usually given an oxytocic drug prophylactically following subsequent deliveries. This question has a false response stem. Look for a CONTRAINDICATION.*
4. ***Correct! Methergine is contraindicated prior to the delivery of the placenta. Great thinking!***

98. A client is receiving propranolol (Inderal) for anxiety. In reviewing the client's discharge plans, the nurse needs to emphasize that:

1. Inderal should be discontinued by gradually tapering it off over time.
2. Inderal should not be taken during pregnancy.
3. Inderal is contraindicated for clients with asthma.
4. Inderal is a safe medication with no known adverse effects.

1. ***Correct. Rapid withdrawal from Inderal in cardiac clients has been associated with cardiac arrhythmias and sudden death. As a general rule, it is discontinued by gradually tapering it off over time, to avoid any adverse responses.***

2. *This is a possibility, but it is not the best option. Most medications should be avoided during pregnancy, but there is no indication that the client in this question is contemplating childbearing or is even female. "Reading in" as simple a fact as gender can lead you astray! There are many facts that, added to this question, could affect the nurse's priority in discharge teaching. Which option deals with a priority that can be true for every client on Inderal?*
3. *This is a true statement, but it is not the best response to this question about discharge teaching. The client's physical health was evaluated prior to starting Inderal to rule out any contraindications. There is a more important point for the nurse to emphasize prior to the client's discharge.*
4. *Wrong. Inderal is a relatively safe medication, but it does have adverse effects.*

99. A 55-year-old client has been taking trifluoperazine (Stelazine) for five years to control her paranoid thoughts. When the client's brother comes to visit, he tells the nurse that he believes all psychiatric medications are a form of "chemical mind control." The nurse's best response to the brother will incorporate which information about antipsychotic medications?

1. They act directly on specific neurotransmitters in the brain to control the client's psychotic symptoms.
2. They act to sedate the client so she cannot engage in behavior that will cause difficulty for either herself or others.
3. They are a cure for psychotic disorders, like schizophrenic reactions, and are therefore an important part of his sister's treatment plan.
4. They have been in use for close to 30 years and are safe and effective drugs for clients who have problems like his sister's.

1. ***Correct. The specific mechanisms of action are still unknown, but research indicates that antipsychotics act directly on the dopamine receptors in the brain and thereby control many target symptoms of psychosis.***
2. *This is partially correct. Antipsychotic drugs do sedate the client to some degree, but that is not their primary mode of action. Look again at the other options to select one that provides a better rationale.*
3. *Incorrect. There is no known cure for schizophrenic disorders at this time. Many clients with these diagnoses have a chronic illness. Treatment is focused on helping them attain their highest level of functioning using medication and psychosocial therapies.*
4. *Although this is true, it is not the best rationale for the nurse to use in responding to the client's concern. Look over the options to select a better rationale.*

100. Which measure would the nurse select as providing the most accurate determination of renal impairment secondary to administration of amphotericin B (Fungizone)?

1. Intake and output.
2. Daily weights.
3. Serum creatinine levels.
4. Serial potassium levels.

1. *No, this would not be the best means to determine renal function. Monitoring input and output can give clues to renal function but cannot accurately define the problem.*
2. *Incorrect. Daily weights are not the best indicator of renal function, although they do serve as a monitoring tool for fluid volume status. Try again.*
3. ***Excellent! Measurement of serum creatinine is used to detect impaired renal function. Serum creatinine should be monitored every other day as the dosage of amphotericin B is increased to optimal level, and then weekly until the drug is discontinued. If serum creatinine increases to 3 mg/ml, the dosage of should be decreased or discontinued until renal function improves.***
4. *No, there is another option that would give an earlier and more accurate clue to decreased renal function.*

Additional Study Materials for NCLEX-RN Candidates

BOOKS

[ ] The Comprehensive NCLEX-RN Review (with disk) $29.95
[ ] The Complete Question and Answer Book for the NCLEX-RN (with disk) $29.95
[ ] Successful Problem-Solving and Test-Taking (with disk) $29.95
[ ] Successful Problem-Solving and Test-Taking (with companion audio tape and disk) $39.95

AUDIOS

[ ] Everything You Need to Know about the NCLEX-RN 32 Tapes *(Save $197)* $249.00
[ ] Tape 1: How to Study for the NCLEX/CAT-RN Exam $13.95
[ ] Tape 2: Assesing lab Values $13.95
[ ] Tape 3: Nutrition $13.95
[ ] Tape 4: Growth and Development $13.95
[ ] Tape 5: Fluids and Electrolytes $13.95

[ ] Module 1: Medical-Surgical $119.00
[ ] Tape 6: Cardiovascular Disorders (M/S Pt 1) $13.95
[ ] Tape 7: Respiratory Disorders (M/S Pt 2) $13.95
[ ] Tape 8: Endocrine Disorders (M/S Pt 3) $13.95
[ ] Tape 9: Blood Disorders (M/S Pt 4) $13.95
[ ] Tape 10: GI/Hepatic/Pancreatic (M/S Pt 5) $13.95
[ ] Tape 11: Renal Disorders (M/S Pt 6) $13.95
[ ] Tape 12: Musculoskeletal (M/S Pt 7) $13.95
[ ] Tape 13: Neurological (M/S Pt 8) $13.95
[ ] Tape 14: Neurological (M/S Pt 9) $13.95
[ ] Tape 15: Questions and Answers (M/S Pt 10) $13.95

[ ] Module 2: Psychiatric $34.95
[ ] Tape 16: Psycho-Social Component (Psy Pt 1) $13.95
[ ] Tape 17: Psychiatric Disorders (Pt. 1) (Psy Pt 2) $13.95
[ ] Tape 18: Psychiatric Disorders (Pt. 2) (Psy Pt 3) $13.95

[ ] Module 3: Maternity $44.95
[ ] Tape 19: Normal Pregnancy (OB Pt 1) $13.95
[ ] Tape 20: Complications of Pregnancy (Pt. 1) (OB Pt 2) ... $13.95
[ ] Tape 21: Complications of Pregnancy (Pt. 2) (OB Pt 3) ... $13.95
[ ] Tape 22: The Newborn (OB Pt 4) $13.95
[ ] Tape 23: Pharmacology* $13.95
[ ] Tape 24: Math and Calculations $13.95
[ ] Tape 25: Emergencies $13.95

[ ] Module 4: Pediatric $44.95
[ ] Tape 26: Pediatric Bacterial (Ped Pt 1) $13.95
[ ] Tape 27: Pediatric Viral (Ped Pt 2) $13.95
[ ] Tape 28: Pediatric Chronic (Ped Pt 3) $13.95
[ ] Tape 29: Pediatric Surgical (Ped Pt 4) $13.95
[ ] Tape 30: Post-Operative Positioning and Tubes $13.95
[ ] Tape 31: The Aging Client $13.95
[ ] Tape 32: Communicable Disease $13.95

VIDEOS

[ ] The Comprehensive NCLEX-RN Video Review 35 Tape Set (*Save $453*) $595.00

[ ] **Module 1: Medical-Surgical Nursing $249.00
[ ] Video 1: Fluids and Electrolytes (M/S Pt 1) $29.95
[ ] Video 2: Respiratory Disorders (Pt 1) (M/S Pt 2) $29.95
[ ] Video 3: Respiratory Disorders (Pt 2) (M/S Pt 3) $29.95
[ ] Video 4: Pre and Post Operative Care (M/S Pt 4) $29.95
[ ] Video 5: GI, Hepatic/Pancreatic (Pt 1) (M/S Pt 5) $29.95
[ ] Video 6: GI, Hepatic/Pancreatic (Pt 2) (M/S Pt 6) $29.95
[ ] Video 7: Musculoskeletal (M/S Pt 7) $29.95
[ ] Video 8: Blood Disorders (M/S Pt 8) $29.95
[ ] Video 9: Endocrine Disorders (M/S Pt 9) $29.95
[ ] Video 10: Cardiovascular Disorders (M/S Pt 10) $29.95
[ ] Video 11: Genitourinary Disorders (M/S Pt 11) $29.95
[ ] Video 12: Neurological Disorders (Pt 1) (M/S Pt 12) $29.95
[ ] Video 13: Neurological Disorders (Pt 2) (M/S Pt 13) $29.95
[ ] Video 14: Oncology Nursing & Burns (M/S Pt 14) $29.95

[ ] **Module 2: Psychiatric Nursing $149.00
[ ] Video 15: Psychiatric Nursing (Psy Pt 1) $29.95
[ ] Video 16: Defense Mechanisms (Psy Pt 2) $29.95
[ ] Video 17: Anxiety Disorders (Psy Pt 3) $29.95
[ ] Video 18: Schizophrenia (Psy Pt 4) $29.95
[ ] Video 19: Mood Disorders (Psy Pt 5) $29.95
[ ] Video 20: Chemical Dependency (Psy Pt 6) $29.95
[ ] Video 21: OMS, Eating, Violence, Legal (Psy Pt 7) $29.95

[ ] **Module 3: Maternity Nursing $149.00
[ ] Video 22: Female Reproductive Nursing (OB Pt 1) $29.95
[ ] Video 23: Labor and Delivery (OB Pt 2) $29.95
[ ] Video 24: Postpartal Adaptation (OB Pt 3) $29.95
[ ] Video 25: Reproductive Risks (OB Pt 4) $29.95
[ ] Video 26: Newborn/High Risk Newborn (OB Pt 5) $29.95
[ ] Video 27: Gynecology (OB Pt 6) $29.95

[ ] **Module 4: Pediatrics Nursing $149.00
[ ] Video 28: Growth and Development (Pt 1) (Ped Pt 1) $29.95
[ ] Video 29: Growth and Development (Pt 2) (Ped Pt 2) $29.95
[ ] Video 30: Children with Anomalie (Ped Pt 3) $29.95
[ ] Video 31: Children with Acute Illness (Ped Pt 4) $29.95
[ ] Video 32: Child Surgical Care (Ped Pt 5) $29.95
[ ] Video 33: Children As Accident Victims (Ped Pt 6) $29.95
[ ] Video 34: Children with Chronic Problem (Ped Pt 7) $29.95
[ ] Video 35: Oncological /Infectious Diseases (Ped Pt 8) $29.95

Core Concept Videos:
[ ] Video 36: Nutrition (Study Guide Not Included) $29.95
[ ] Video 37: Pharmacology $29.95

SOFTWARE

[ ] Order both Q&A and Pharmacology Q&A $219.00
[ ] Steps to Success for the NCLEX-RN Exam $69.00
[ ] The Q&A Software Review for the NCLEX-RN $149.00
[ ] The Q&A Pharmacology Review for the NCLEX-RN $89.00

* Includes a study guide.
** Includes *The Comprehensive NCLEX-RN Review* book.

Call, Fax, or Mail Order to MEDS, Inc.
See order form on next page.

MEDS, INC.
Excellence in Nursing Education

SPECIAL TIPS FOR USING THE COMPANION COMPUTER DISK

If you do not own a personal computer, be sure to inquire whether the learning lab in your nursing program has computers that you can use! You will not want to miss this opportunity to practice using the NCLEX computer format.

No special computer skills are required for using the companion diskette provided with this book. Just follow the instructions for inserting the diskette. Then, be sure to select the helpful section on "How to Use This Program."

The companion diskette includes 100 test questions in NCLEX format. It also includes a choice of two modes of operation: Simulation Test Mode, and Practice Test Mode. We suggest that you select Simulation Test Mode first.

In **Simulation Test Mode,** you will have the opportunity to take the test in a format simulating the NCLEX and under NCLEX exam conditions. ***NOTE:*** In the NCLEX, you cannot skip questions, and you cannot go back and change your answer in a question once the computer has moved on to the next question. So it is very important to try out your test-taking skills in NCLEX Simulation Test Mode!

At the end of the simulation test, you will receive your score, a readout on the amount of time you required to complete the exam, and a Personal Performance Analysis. Finally, this special MEDS, Inc. program also lets you go back and view the questions that you answered incorrectly. Be sure to use these superior program features!

Next, we recommend that you select the **Practice Test Mode.** This is the MEDS, Inc. special format for NCLEX candidates, specially designed for maximum learning in a Q&A context. Practice Test Mode features instant, color-coded feedback about whether your answer is right or wrong, plus a complete explanation of *why* that option is *or is not* the best option. In Practice Test Mode, you may select one option after another in each question and instantly view the rationale for each option. The superb rationales incorporate detailed nursing knowledge, problem solving strategies to increase your critical thinking skills, and test-taking tips using MEDS proven test-taking strategies.

You may use the companion diskette as many times as you wish. The answers you select are not permanently entered into the program, just recorded and scored. You may wish to return to the Simulation Test Mode again after studying the questions in the Practice Test Mode, to review the information you have learned and practice using your test-taking strategies.

We are sure that you will find this diskette to be a powerful tool in your NCLEX review plan. For more practice in a computerized testing environment, MEDS, Inc. publishes a superb Q&A computer series, which also features both the Simulation Test Mode and Practice Test Mode. In addition, MEDS, Inc. also offers a unique tutorial on test-taking strategies and other computer learning tools for the NCLEX candidate. For more information, please call MEDS, Inc. at (301) 622-9191. We are always pleased to assist you!